PRAI…

Love Life Sober

"With honesty, curiosity, and the up-close familiar tone of a trusted friend, Osborne pulls the curtain back on the easily overlooked devastation caused by substance addiction. But she doesn't stop there. Her story demonstrates that when you actively engage your heart in the vulnerable process of healing, the very struggles that once held you down can become a lifeline of freedom to others."

—Christopher Cook, author of *Healing What You Can't Erase* and podcast host of *Win Today with Christopher Cook*

"*Love Life Sober* is a masterful, transformative, and grace-filled guide for any woman who wants to put the cork in the bottle—and leave it there. In this deeply compassionate book, Christy Osborne blends spiritual wisdom with forty days of actionable strategies, empowering you to embrace sobriety with faith and resilience. There is no condemnation here, only grace and a refreshing one-day-at-a-time approach that will give you back the vibrant life you were created for."

—Jennifer Dukes Lee, author of *Growing Slow* and *It's All Under Control*

"There are very few books that, just a few pages in, I am absolutely certain will change lives, and this is one of them. I cannot overstate the importance of this book. On a topic that is so often mired in shame, Osborne overflows with compassion and grace. If you are ready to reset your relationship with alcohol, *Love Life Sober* is for you."

—Sharon Hodde Miller, author of *The Cost of Control: Why We Crave It, the Anxiety It Gives Us, and the Real Power God Promises*

"Christy Osborne is so relatable as she shares her story of partnering with God to let go of the wine glass in exchange for real freedom! These forty days provide a road map through the twists and turns of the sober-curious journey. Through practical insights and biblical wisdom, you'll feel supported and know you are not alone. I'm so grateful Osborne has brought her faith into the conversation, as we need more Christian women speaking into this alcohol-centric culture."

—Jenn Kautsch, founder of Sober Sis and author of *Look Alive, Sis*

"As a mental health pioneer, I am thrilled to see Christy Osborne bring her invaluable work to the world. In *Love Life Sober,* she masterfully intertwines mental health and sobriety, showcasing the profound transformation that comes from renewing one's mind. By tackling the mental patterns linked to alcohol use, she leads readers to a healthier, more balanced mindset, infused with truth and gratitude. Osborne's approach powerfully demonstrates that overcoming alcohol dependency is a crucial step toward enhanced mental well-being and a deeply fulfilling life."

—Christy Boulware, author of *Nervous Breakthrough* and founder of Fearless Unite

"*Love Life Sober* is a breath of fresh air! I love how Christy Osborne boldly, yet compassionately, guides women toward honest reflection around the everyday addictions we all grapple with in our fast-paced world. This book not only sheds fresh light on the real risks of alcohol use but also offers practical tips to help readers walk the path of freedom and deepen their relationship with God. It is a must-read!"

—Ali Kennedy, MTh, PCC, author, speaker, coach, minister in the international church

"In an era when wellness and mindfulness have become central to personal development, Christy Osborne presents a timely and transformative guide with *Love Life Sober.* This forty-day fast is not just a book but an invitation to a journey that promises to rejuvenate your spirit and renew your mind. Thank you, Christy Osborne, for bringing faith into the conversation around alcohol. It's not only refreshing but necessary."

—Karla Adkins, co-owner of The Zero Proof Life and author of *And She Came Tumbling Down*

"This book is going to help so many women who, like me, were feeling stuck in the clutches of something they couldn't figure out how to control. When I first started working with Christy Osborne, I knew I was drinking more than I wanted to, but I didn't recognize how alcohol was separating me from God. I'd always called myself a Christian but was burned-out, anxious, and exhausted. Through Osborne's coaching, podcast, and friendship, she led me back to the Lord."

—Lauren, Love Life Sober coaching client

"Friends, I have searched the world of literature over, and there is truly nothing like this forty-day journey with Christy Osborne. With her feet firmly planted in God's Word, she is candid, warm, laid-back, and brilliant as she breaks down the neuroscience behind why we drink, leads us to examine ourselves without judgment, and teaches us how we can say goodbye to alcohol for as long as we like. *Love Life Sober* is a devotional, memoir, and handbook all in one, packed with tools that helped me give up alcohol for good. Best of all, there is not a drop of shame or condemnation in it—only freedom and grace! I will always keep a spare copy on hand, using it to help any sister in Christ live a life of freedom, paid for by Jesus on the cross."

—Brittany, Love Life Sober coaching client

"This book made me feel seen and supported, like I had a trusted friend by my side. Christy Osborne writes with compassion and understanding about the struggles Christian women face with alcohol. *Love Life Sober* is a must-read for anyone seeking to reclaim their life."

—Ashley, Love Life Sober coaching client

"*Love Life Sober* is a groundbreaking guide that seamlessly integrates science, coaching, and Scripture, offering an empowering path to freedom from alcohol. Osborne's unwavering encouragement, infectious positivity, and practical expertise create a nurturing and motivational environment, making this transformative journey both attainable and inspiring. Her clear and insightful explanations of how alcohol affects our brains and bodies provide essential knowledge that every woman should have. This book is a must-read for anyone seeking to reclaim their joy, improve their mental health, and deepen their relationship with Jesus."

—Kristen Dalton, former Miss USA
and author of *The Sparkle Effect*

"*Love Life Sober* is a game changer for those looking to break free from the cycle of alcohol dependence. Osborne's insightful guidance, combined with a deep understanding of the science behind alcohol's impact on our bodies, offers a clear path to better health and well-being. By shedding light on how alcohol disrupts sleep and fuels anxiety, Osborne empowers women to reclaim their rest and find genuine peace."

—William Porter, author of
Alcohol Explained and *Alcohol Explained 2*

LOVE LIFE SOBER

Love · Life · Sober

A 40-DAY
ALCOHOL FAST TO
REDISCOVER
YOUR JOY,
IMPROVE YOUR
HEALTH,
AND RENEW
YOUR MIND

Christy Osborne

FOREWORD BY WENDY SPEAKE

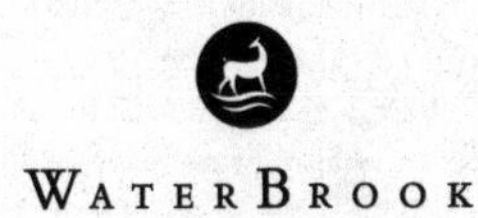

Italics in Scripture quotations reflect the author's added emphasis.

Details in some anecdotes and stories have been changed to protect the identities of the persons involved.

A WaterBrook Trade Paperback Original

Published in the United States by WaterBrook, an imprint of Random House, a division of Penguin Random House LLC.

LIBRARY OF CONGRESS CATALOGING-IN-PUBLICATION DATA
Names: Osborne, Christy, author.
Title: Love life sober : a 40 day alcohol fast to rediscover your joy, improve your health, and renew your mind / Christy Osborne.
Description: Colorado Springs : WaterBrook, 2024. | "A WaterBrook trade paperback original." | Includes bibliographical references. | Summary: "A 40-day, alcohol-free journey to reset drinking habits, reconnect with yourself, and strengthen your relationship with Jesus from a certified sobriety coach with you-can-do-it positivity"— Provided by publisher.
Identifiers: LCCN 2024008379 | ISBN 9780593600733 (trade paperback) | ISBN 9780593600740 (ebook)
Subjects: LCSH: Temperance and religion. | Temperance—Religious aspects—Christianity. | Alcoholism—Prevention.
Classification: LCC HV5187 .O74 2024 | DDC 261.8/32292—dc23/eng/20240515
LC record available at https://lccn.loc.gov/2024008379

Printed in the United States of America on acid-free paper

waterbrookmultnomah.com

1st Printing

Book design by Barbara M. Bachman

For Chris, Ella, and Carter.
I thank God for you three every single morning.

And for my mom.
I can't wait to tell you all about
what happened after you left for heaven.

Foreword

I'M THE GIRL WHO WRITES BOOKS NOBODY ELSE WOULD CHOOSE to write. Surprisingly, the more uncomfortable the topic and the more I'd prefer to avoid the conversation altogether, the more books I sell on those topics. I talk about mommy anger and sugar addiction and all the icky things we'd rather keep hidden away behind closed doors—and certainly not share in lovely little squares on Instagram. That said, there is one particularly private stone I have not publicly turned over, allowing the light of God's Word to illuminate it and lead into freedom. Of course, you know which stone I'm talking about: alcohol.

After launching the book *The 40-Day Sugar Fast* in 2019, I became very aware that a forty-day alcohol fast was desperately needed, but the door never opened for me to write about it, no matter how hard I knocked. Which is why I am beyond thrilled to lift my mocktail and toast Christy Osborne for her courage and creativity in writing *Love Life Sober*.

Bringing secret struggles out into the light takes great courage—not just for authors but also for readers. So, I raise my metaphorical glass and acknowledge your courage too!

During one of my annual online sugar fasts, I spoke to a brave woman who told me about the day she realized she had a sincere addiction to sugar. She had found freedom from alcohol after years of being stuck in the drinking cycle. One day, she realized she was hiding her stash of sugar in all the same places where she used to hide bottles of wine. In a cowboy boot in her closet, she kept a box of girl-scout cookies; beneath the bathroom sink and behind rolls of toilet paper, she hid a stash of chocolate-covered almonds; and in the hard-to-get-to cabinet above the fridge, she tucked away out of sight the bag of mismatched holiday candies. In the same way she once reached up to take hold of a bottle of wine in the mid-afternoon, she now retrieved her sweets. She'd gone from self-medicating with one substance to another.

As she shared her story with me, I pictured her there in her kitchen, reaching up for a bottle of wine or a box of treats, and suggested that the answer to any and all struggles can only be found when we reach *just a little bit higher.* The One who reigns above all the stresses and sorrows of this life is enthroned above our refrigerators too. "Reach a little higher" became my battle cry when leading ladies into these very private fights.

Whether you are reaching for alcohol, sugar, or social media, or streaming shows to make it through your days, I invite you to reach a little higher these next forty days. Set your eyes on the One who invited His disciples and invites us: "Come to me, all you who are weary and burdened, and I will give you rest" (Matthew 11:28).

You are so brave, and I am cheering you on!

—Wendy Speake

Author of THE 40-DAY SUGAR FAST, THE 40-DAY SOCIAL MEDIA FAST, *and* TRIGGERS

Contents

Introduction

MARCH 9, 2020. I WAKE UP WITH A HEADACHE, PAR FOR the course over the last two years. I reach over and grab my phone to check the time while keeping one eye closed. I still have on yesterday's makeup. It isn't even the makeup from the night before; it's makeup from lunch at a little Italian restaurant in Clapham, where we celebrated my children turning eight and ten with close friends.

I take a second to rate the category of my hangover. Darn. It's a bad one. I immediately try to think of what I must do today and when I can lie down again. It's a Monday morning. I'm used to this predicament because I face it routinely: Mondays mean I have to get the children to school. But I can come home and nap after that—all alone, in an empty house. I can nurse my hangover in peace.

I pick up my phone and see a text from my cousin Katie in Los Angeles: "Missing our beloved Terry. I love you. [Heart emoji]" My heart sinks into my stomach, and I feel like I might vomit. Terry—my mom. Today marks the second anniversary of her death.

My cousin's message isn't the only one that has popped up, but I don't feel like responding to even my closest friends' condolences. They don't understand how I'm feeling. How could they? They all have their moms still. The loneliness overwhelms me. I put my phone back on my nightstand and roll over, hoping my husband, Chris, will volunteer to take the children to school this morning.

I spend most of the day in bed, wallowing in grief. I scroll through social media and try to distract myself with Netflix, but mainly I just feel sorry for myself. The hangover is real, my stomach is churning, and my only aim is to just get through this awful day. I purposely ignore anyone calling to check on me, and when flowers arrive from Chris in the afternoon, I want to roll my eyes. The beautiful pink and red bouquet from my favorite florist in Chelsea won't bring back my mom, so what's the point?

Two. Years.

What had I done in the past two years? Absolutely nothing. It felt like I just had been drinking—drinking, drinking, drinking.

I look back on my Instagram posts from the last two years. How did I look so happy when I was so sad and broken? There are photos of my trips to Ibiza, Saint-Tropez, and Paris. Skiing in the Italian Alps. A photo of me at brunch with Posh Spice herself; I have a big smile on my face. *How?*

I eventually scroll back to posts from 2018, right after my mom died—the royal wedding. Sky News, the UK-based news network, needed a peppy American to cover the wedding who could represent the excitement people felt in the USA. I watch my interviews from that time. I should've been given an Emmy for appearing that happy on screen when I was so miserable inside. There were so many days like this when I didn't want to get out of bed. There are comments on the post that say things like, "Your mom would be so proud."

As we all know, Instagram is zero reflection of reality. So, what had my life really looked like in the past two years? It looked like waking up with a headache, planning what I had to do to get through the day, hoping there was a lunch in my calendar so there was an excuse to have a glass (or three) of cold white wine at noon, and, if there wasn't a lunch, trying to get to the afternoon as quickly as possible so I could open up a bottle of wine when the homework books came out after school.

Everything looked so glossy and pretty on the surface. But it just wasn't. When the afternoon wine bottle popped open, I felt relief. I could go fuzzy again. I didn't have to handle all the painful stuff. I didn't have to think about the fact that I wasn't being a great mom. I didn't have to think about my collapsing marriage to Chris. I didn't have to think about how I didn't have a mom anymore, that my children no longer had their "Grammie." The wine became a total and complete escape for two years.

Two. Years.

I wonder where I will be in another two years if I keep drinking like this? My mind pings back and forth between *Oh, come on, I'm fine. Not one person has called me out on my drinking,* and *This has to stop*.

Then, in an attempt to shut up the internal battle in my head, I quite literally shout to God, "Jesus, I can't do this anymore!"

I certainly don't want to look or feel like this anymore. I don't want to spend every March 9 for the rest of my life nursing a hangover and hiding in my dark bedroom. I need this day to mean something else. And so, on March 9, 2020, in honor of my mom, I decide to try to be better for my little family—and to take a break from alcohol.

. . .

IN THE FOLLOWING DAYS AND MONTHS, I STRUGGLED TO REmain alcohol-free. I battled cravings and felt terrified to tell friends what I was doing. I didn't have one friend who didn't drink. I worried my social life would suffer. I had no idea how to navigate life without alcohol. I felt scared and alone.

I kept returning to 2 Corinthians 12:9, which says, " 'My grace is sufficient for you, for my power is made perfect in weakness.' Therefore I will boast all the more gladly about my weaknesses, so that Christ's power may rest on me." God's power was made evident to me in my weakness around alcohol. He would take this struggle of mine and turn it into something I could never have imagined. Verse 10 says, "That is why, for Christ's sake, I delight in weaknesses. . . . For when I am weak, then I am strong." When I finally surrendered to God, I felt more powerful than ever before because of His work in me. I knew I had a story and a message to share with other women struggling with alcohol.

Throughout my drinking days, I constantly prayed to Jesus, asking for His help. I now know He was with me during my darkest days and had a significant plan for me. He heard my prayers, and I felt His presence. The year I let go of alcohol, I researched everything I could about alcohol use disorder and addiction while also growing closer to Jesus than I had ever been. Finally, I felt God call me to be vocal about my sobriety journey, and so I did just that. I started documenting my day-to-day learning on my Instagram during Covid lockdowns. It was scary to be that open and vulnerable, but the response I got was overwhelming. So many friends, old and new, reached out and asked how I had found freedom from alcohol. I tried to help in any way I could and recommended books, podcasts, and resources that had helped me.

I felt God nudging me to explore more ways to help others, so at the end of 2020 I enrolled in my first life coaching certification program with a focus on sobriety. I've since become certified in multiple programs and have been blessed with a flourishing private coaching practice where I get to support women around the world.

Coaching is all about listening and allowing another person the space to discuss their struggles. As I listened and asked thoughtful questions over the past few years, I heard from ladies who had also lost their faith or felt far from Jesus due to their drinking. I longed to create a resource that combined practical coaching based on neuroscience with biblical support and encouragement. God has blessed me with making that dream a reality through this book.

I am excited to spend the next forty days with you on this alcohol fast that is packed with grace, compassion, and a sprinkle of science. I know taking a break from alcohol is hard, and it can seem overwhelming. I've been right where you are. But the fantastic news I have for you is that Jesus is with you right now and will show up for you, just like He did for me.

If you stick with this alcohol fast for the next forty days, you may experience some incredible benefits, including better sleep, brighter skin, improved hydration, and reduced brain fog. Damage to your stomach lining will repair itself. You may also decrease your cancer risk, reduce your resting heart rate, lower your cholesterol, and improve your blood pressure. You will give a healthy boost to your liver and gut health. You will save tons of time, money, and energy.

My hope is that you will also feel closer to Jesus. Being stuck in the drinking cycle put a barrier between me and God. When I started my own fast and began to make space for Him with a clear head, my spiritual life transformed. The ability to pray with a sober mind, to take time to meditate on His Word, and to surrender my disordered drinking to Him brought us closer than ever.

God made us all so different, but if you're anything like me, after forty days of not drinking you will feel better than you've felt in years and your relationship with Jesus will take on a whole new meaning. I'm so excited for you.

I'd love to connect with you and cheer you on. If you're documenting your journey on Instagram, make sure to tag @lovelifesoberwithchristy and use #LoveLifeSober40DayFast. I've also created a celebration tracker so you can have a visual representation of how far you've come. You can find your personal tracker at lovelifesober40dayfast.com.

LOVE LIFE SOBER

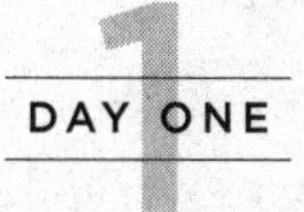

DAY ONE

Starting with Grace

I sought the Lord, *and he answered me;*
he delivered me from all my fears.
Those who look to him are radiant;
their faces are never covered with shame.

—PSALM 34:4–5

WELCOME TO YOUR FORTY-DAY ALCOHOL FAST! EVERY morning that I've sat down to write this book, I've prayed God would use my story and the lessons I've learned to encourage you. The goal of this book is to help you decide how big of a role you want alcohol to play in your life. Maybe you know it's time to give up for good because you already know alcohol is taking more than it's giving. Or perhaps you only drink a few times a week, but you've realized your sleep and energy levels are suffering and you need a reset. Whatever your reason, you've picked up this book because a part of you knows it's time to take a break from booze.

First, I want to celebrate this moment with you. You've taken the very first step of becoming aware. Your eyes are open. You're aware that alcohol may not be serving you anymore, and that awareness has led you to take a big action step: opening this book. You're on your way to better physical, mental, and spiritual health, stronger relationships, and so much more. This is a big move, and I'm so proud of you.

Let's start with a few fundamental principles to prepare us for the journey ahead.

SHUT THE TRAPDOOR

During the next forty days, commit to not drinking alcohol. Here is a visual that I love to use with my clients. Imagine you have a little trapdoor in the back of your brain, an escape hatch of sorts. If that little door is open, you will choose alcohol because it's the easy-button answer that you are used to. But if you shut that trapdoor, you've taken alcohol off the table for the next forty days. You are making the conscious choice not to drink. This might be a good time to get the alcohol out of the house if you feel like it may be too tempting to have it so accessible.

GROWTH POINTS

Try to stick with the fast for forty consecutive days so that you can start feeling better. (That's why we're here, to get you to feel your best.) However, if you do have a drink at any time during the forty-day fast, don't think of it as a slipup or failure. Think of it as a growth point. You are here to learn and grow.

If these growth points happen, don't stop or reset your fast. Instead, take out your journal and consider the following questions:

- Why did you decide to drink? (Was it a particularly stressful morning? Did something happen at work

that overwhelmed you? Was your teenager extra spicy with you?)
- How did you feel in the hours immediately after drinking? How did you feel the next morning?
- What can you learn from this?

Even though growth points can make you feel like you've failed, they are a hugely important part of this journey. Don't fall into the shame trap; instead, get curious and figure out what exactly happened so that you can make a different decision the next time. Think of a little toddler learning to walk. If he falls, do we shout at him and say, "You're a failure! You must have a serious problem; you can't even walk!" No, of course not! We pick him up and say, "You're doing a great job, little guy. Try again." He's learning. Growing. Trying something new and becoming aware of what works and what doesn't. And so are you. This is about grace, compassion, and curiosity.

MAKE THE TIME

Set aside time every single day to complete your daily reading. Piggyback it onto your quiet time or morning routine. Or if you need something to fill the five o'clock wine witching hour, read it then. You will have new information to think about and helpful questions to ask yourself. I recommend revisiting the Bible verses we reference throughout the book and journaling your thoughts and emotions as you read along. The more you put into the next forty days, the more you will get out of it.

AN EXPERIMENTAL MINDSET

You may have done a Dry January or a Sober October before, mustering all your willpower to stay away from alcohol for a month. I did those too. However, when I completed the month, I drank just as much, if not more, afterward. This fast is different. In addition to not drinking, we are going to take the next forty days to learn:

- How alcohol is affecting your life
- Why you sometimes fall into addictive patterns
- Whether or not the assumed benefits of alcohol are even true

If you decide to go back to drinking at the end of these forty days, that is 100 percent your choice. *You* get to decide what kind of role alcohol has in your life. Alcohol will always be around; it's not going anywhere. Most of us know well what it feels like to drink regularly or often. Now's the time to figure out what *not* drinking feels like. This is an experimental reset.

Take one day at a time. You don't have to have the mindset of "I'm never drinking again" right now. And I really don't want you to stress about any parties, vacations, or events in the future, even if they take place in these forty days. Just focus on today. You don't know now how you will feel the day of that event or party; you can cross that bridge when you get to it. As I always say to my clients, there is no point in future-tripping before you even arrive at that date. More importantly, Jesus said in Matthew 6:34, "Do not worry about tomorrow, for tomorrow will worry about itself."

While writing this book, I'm doing a different kind of experiment: a gluten experiment. A few years ago, I learned I have a gluten intolerance. I thought this was horrible news at the time. How could I go the rest of my life without eating bread, pastries, *pasta,* and all the delicious desserts with gluten in them? But I know I don't feel good when I eat gluten, so I decided to go on an experimental reset and try a gluten-free diet. I feel so much better: I no longer get sharp stomach pains, and my digestion has greatly improved.

The key to successfully testing out what my body needs was to approach it from an experimental mindset. I haven't once said, "I'm never eating pasta again." If I wind up in Paris and choose to eat the buttery croissant, I will. But now I am armed with that knowledge of how gluten makes me feel.

I want you to approach this fast like that. You don't have to say forever. Just get curious and be open to learning.

ONE THING AT A TIME

Please don't try to start a diet, completely cut out sugar, or begin a strict exercise routine during the next forty days. Please don't start an intermittent fasting regimen. In fact, you'll want to eat regular meals packed with protein to curb cravings, so please don't try to restrict food right now. We will talk about incorporating joyful movement and handling sugar cravings, but this is not the time to make multiple wellness goals. I have coached so many women who want to simultaneously quit alcohol, lose fifteen pounds, and start working out five times a day. It's too overwhelming, so they burn out quickly. Researchers have found that people who set too many goals for themselves fail at all of them.[1] Baby steps, babe, just like that little toddler.

DOCUMENT YOUR TRANSFORMATION

Today is the first day of your fast. I love a good transformation, and I'm sure you do too. After forty days of not drinking, I witnessed a remarkable change in the appearance of my face. The puffiness diminished and the persistent redness faded to the point where I found myself wearing far less makeup than before because my face was so clear. You, also, will be amazed at the difference in the way you look and feel. I want you to have photographic proof and written evidence of how far you've come. I've seen incredible transformations in just forty days with my clients. Their eyes are clear, and they have more clarity of mind and inner peace. The same and much more is possible for you, my beautiful friend. So snap a selfie right now to document your growth. Take notes, either in the margins of this book or in a separate journal, on each win you experience along this journey. Trust me, you will want to look back at how far you've come.

Use the special celebration tracker I created for you to mark important alcohol-free milestones like your first alcohol-free date, first alcohol-free book club, first alcohol-free wedding, and so many more. Every little step is progress. Head to lovelifesober40dayfast.com to download your copy of the tracker.

YOU DON'T HAVE TO COUNT DAYS

There are lots of apps out there that help you count sober days. Use them if they motivate you. However, *please don't reset the counter* if you have a growth point. If you were running a marathon and tripped at mile twenty-three, would you go back to the starting line? If you have ten days alcohol-free and on the eleventh day you have a growth point, you made it ten days; that's amazing. Don't focus on the one; focus on the ten. And start counting again with day eleven on your next alcohol-free day. Another helpful tool could be printing out a monthly calendar and checking off the days you haven't had a drink. At the end of the month, look at the percentage of days you've not had a drink. If you're drinking 25 percent less than before—that's a win! This is about *progress,* not perfection.

Your personal celebration tracker I mentioned also has a way to mark your forty days of not drinking, even if they're not consecutive.

TiNA

At the end of each reading, I will leave you with TiNA, a Tiny New Action. These simple and practical steps will help you gain momentum on this journey, implement what you are learning, and recognize how life without alcohol makes you feel.

Quite a few of your TiNAs will involve journaling. Don't put too much pressure on yourself with the whole journaling thing. Some women love it, some don't, but the more time you spend thinking (and writing if you can) about the questions I ask you, the more you will learn about yourself.

Today, your TiNA is to take a selfie to document the first day of your alcohol fast.

You're already on your way. Let's do this!

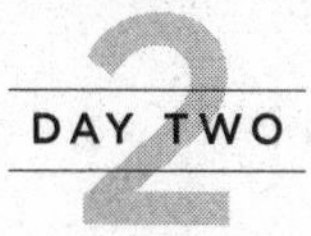

DAY TWO

You're Not Alone

Even when I walk
through the darkest valley . . .
you are close beside me.

—PSALM 23:4, NLT

IN MARCH 2020—WHEN I WAS SICK OF HEADACHES, HORRIble sleep, and feeling anxious all the time—I shouted a desperate prayer: "Jesus, I can't do this anymore!" I knew then that the next several days were going to be very different. I wasn't sure what a life without my nightly wine would look like or how my social life would be affected, but I knew I was ready to feel better. And if anyone could pull me off the nightly wine merry-go-round, it was Jesus.

Even though I had grown up in church, it had been years since I'd had a proper relationship with God. I knew He was there, but my drinking had created a divide between us. However, in that moment of clarity, when I knew I'd had enough, I knew He was the one to cry out to.

At that time, I didn't have one friend who didn't drink. Not one. I remember telling a dear friend that I was taking a break from drinking, and one of the first things she said was, "You're going to need a whole new set of friends."

I felt alone. I felt scared. Wine was my ultimate reward. It was my treat at the end of the day. It was the thing that made everything more fun and made the unenjoyable stuff tolerable. I didn't know how I'd get through. So let me encourage you, babe. Even if you feel alone, you are not alone. You are *not* the only one thinking about drinking less.

A recent study showed that 52 percent of adult Americans are trying to reduce their alcohol intake.[1] That's over half the country. I'd be willing to bet that every person you know has questioned their drinking at one point or another, even if it's just, *I shouldn't have that second glass*. Most women desire to drink less because they know deep down it doesn't make them feel great. If you want proof that drinking is slowly going out of fashion, look to Gen Z. A study in 2018 reported 28 percent of college students said they didn't drink alcohol, which is up from the 20 percent reported in 2002.[2]

A 2022 article in *Vogue* observes: "Has everyone stopped drinking? It certainly feels that way. Over the last year, dozens of my former cocktailers-in-arms have leaped onto the wagon for insufferably sensible aims like preserving their marriages or their health—or at least for an extended annual reset in Dry January or Sober October."[3] You can't be alone in this if even *Vogue* recognizes the health trend, right?

We also see the trend showing up in the number of nonalcoholic beverage sales. According to data from the International Wine and Spirit Research Company, the market value of the no- and low-alcohol category exceeded a staggering $11 billion in 2022, a significant jump from $8 billion in 2018.[4] This shift in consumer preference has also drawn the attention of celebrities such as Katy Perry, Kylie Minogue, and Bella Hadid, who have all ventured into the nonalcoholic beverage market by launching their own products.[5]

If you've been out to a restaurant lately, you've likely seen mocktail menus offered alongside standard alcoholic drinks menus.

So even if you feel like you're the only one in your group of friends, your PTA, or your church thinking about changing their relationship with alcohol, I want you to know that you're not alone. The tide is turning, and more and more women are trying to drink less.

JOURNEY WITH JESUS

Most importantly, you are not alone during these forty days (and beyond) because you've got Jesus. He is with you here right now as you're reading this. As Paul wrote in Romans 5:3–4, "We know that suffering produces perseverance; perseverance, character; and character, hope." Yes, this may be hard, but it also might change your life and teach you incredible lessons about how God can show up for you. As soon as I asked Him to help me, to be with me, and to go on this journey with me, I didn't feel alone anymore. The power of the Holy Spirit gives us peace that surpasses our understanding (Philippians 4:7, ESV).

God also has a plan for you. He already knows how this journey is going to turn out for you. It may just bring you closer to God and your family, as it did for me.

Invite Him to join you on this journey. Take a minute to say a simple prayer and ask Him for wisdom, strength, and direction. Go on, close your eyes real quick and do this now.

SET A FEELINGS-BASED GOAL

In the beginning stages of my own alcohol fast, I asked myself one question each morning: *How do I want to feel today?*

Almost everything we do, we do to *feel* a certain way. We buy new shoes because of the way we'll feel wearing them. Even certain tasks we may not want to do, like filing our taxes or going to the dentist, give us the feeling of being financially secure and healthy. It's much easier to adjust our behavior when we know how we want to feel. Remember when I told you about my gluten experiment? My goal wasn't to cut out gluten forever but to feel better and see if cutting out gluten would help.

Likewise, you may have picked up this book with the goal of drinking less, but I urge you to reframe your goal into a feelings-based one. For instance, you might aspire to feel better, achieve better sleep, or have more energy. By adopting this approach, your goal becomes about enhancing your well-being rather than simply depriving yourself. It also allows for clear measurement, as you'll know when you've achieved your goal. If you're feeling better, that's a clear win. However, if your goal solely revolves around drinking "less," it can be challenging to determine what "less" truly means. Let's shift our focus to the power of feeling better.

TiNA

IN YOUR JOURNAL, WRITE DOWN YOUR FEELINGS-based goals. Write how you want to feel each day for the rest of this fast. More energized? More patient? More joyful? More clearheaded? Take this one step further and write your feelings-based goal on a sticky note for your bathroom mirror or make it the background on your phone. It will remind you of the real reason you're walking this journey.

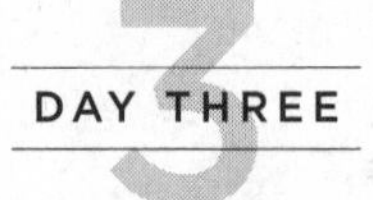

DAY THREE

Rock Bottom Not Required

> *But he said to me, "My grace is sufficient for you, for my power is made perfect in weakness." Therefore I will boast all the more gladly about my weaknesses, so that Christ's power may rest on me.*
>
> —2 CORINTHIANS 12:9

I'LL NEVER FORGET A CONVERSATION I HAD ONE DAY WHILE standing in line at the school gates, waiting to pick up my two kids, Ella and Carter, from school. A mom I knew relatively well stood beside me. It was the first week school was open since Covid had hit. I had been vocal about my sobriety journey on Instagram, and clearly, this mom had seen what I had been up to. "Oh my gosh," she said. "You didn't like, have a *problem* . . . did you?"

I stared at her, taken aback.

The questions came tumbling out of her. "How much were you drinking? Every night? But I've never seen you drunk, ever."

I responded with something like, "I was drinking enough to want to stop drinking. It didn't make me feel good anymore."

Her line of questioning took me back to the late nights when I would sit googling rehab centers and wellness retreats.

Did my drinking warrant rehab, or was it more of a wellness detox that I needed? I had no idea where I fell on the spectrum, but it didn't feel close enough to rock bottom yet. After all, I hadn't had a DUI, my marriage was still intact, and my kids seemed okay. My conclusion that my drinking wasn't "bad enough" to warrant needing outside help almost gave me a kind of permission to keep drinking as I was, even though I knew deep down it wasn't serving me anymore. I had this niggling feeling that God was calling me to more and that alcohol was standing in the way of living my best life for Him.

Recently, I had a coaching call with a lovely lady, Jan, who told me how exhausted she was. She never could stop at one drink. After too much wine, she became cruel to her husband and short with her children. And then she added, "But I haven't had a rock bottom or anything. So maybe I don't need to stop drinking yet."

I could relate to every word Jan said. But why do we wait for it to get worse? Why do we believe that drinking must cost us more than it already has before we can justify taking a break?

I went to my doctor recently for my forty-year-old checkup. I hadn't seen her in a while, so I told her about my sobriety journey and coaching practice during our appointment. She looked at me, confused, and asked the same thing

the mom at the school gates did. "But, wait, did you have a problem?" This time, I was even more perplexed. This was my doctor questioning me, and I thought giving up alcohol was a wise decision even if solely just for the health benefits. How much of a "problem" did it need to be?

The following week, I tried a new chiropractor and had

the same conversation yet again. I was shocked. Why did even some medical professionals seem to believe that drinking needed to reach a certain level of unmanageability to be addressed? (You'll probably share my level of surprise when you've read through day twenty-nine, which is about all the health risks we now know about alcohol.)

Can I encourage you today, my friend? It's not about how bad or how much. It's not about rock bottom. You don't need to wait for things to get worse when a better way is available right now. Waiting on a rock-bottom moment prolongs the pain you're currently in, no matter the level of pain that is. But here's the excellent news: The present version of yourself, with God's help, is more than capable of breaking free. He is with you and will sustain and guide you through every single step of this journey. He is mighty in you. His strength is made perfect in your weakness.

THE FRUIT TEST

Instead of counting glasses or waiting for a rock bottom, let's turn to the truth. As Christians, we have been given the gift of the Holy Spirit, whose presence will produce the fruit of the Spirit. Galatians 5:22–23 says, "But the Holy Spirit produces this kind of fruit in our lives: love, joy, peace, patience, kindness, goodness, faithfulness, gentleness, and self-control. There is no law against these things" (NLT).

When I read that passage, I realized wine was getting in the way of my joy and peace. My capacity for patience was laughable; getting horrible sleep meant I was exhausted and never had enough patience for anyone—my children, my husband, the Starbucks barista. I shamed myself constantly for not having enough self-control around wine. So here's my question for you, babe: Is wine stealing your fruit? If so, I would offer that it might be getting in the way of your relationship with Jesus, just like it was for me.

Isn't this a better litmus test than hitting rock bottom as you decide whether or not you need to make a change?

TiNA

STOP COUNTING GLASSES; START COUNTING YOUR fruit. Take a few minutes today and meditate and pray about the fruit of the Spirit. Write out Galatians 5:22–23 in your journal. How has alcohol stifled the growth of each of these attributes?

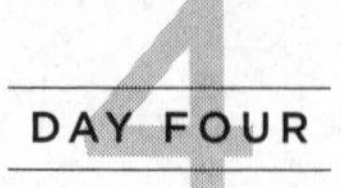

DAY FOUR

Renewing Your Mind

Do not conform to the pattern of this world, but be transformed by the renewing of your mind. Then you will be able to test and approve what God's will is—his good, pleasing and perfect will.

—ROMANS 12:2

FOR A LONG TIME, I IGNORED THE DAMAGE I WAS EXPERIENCING from drinking every night, even if I was drinking *just* a couple of glasses. I thought I should be able to handle the constant feeling of exhaustion and being slightly (sometimes not so slightly) hungover because those feelings become "normal" when you drink all the time. Everyone around me seemed to be able to handle the physical and mental fallout just fine, including my closest girlfriends. No one talked about having a "problem" with alcohol.

I certainly didn't identify with the "alcoholic" label. After all, I wasn't drinking in the mornings and didn't *feel* physically dependent on alcohol. I never got the shakes if I missed a drink. But truthfully, wine, and sometimes tequila, was hindering my relationships, work, energy levels, and physical and mental health. Each day, I would wake up feeling fuzzy, power through while getting the children out the door for school, and then pray to God that I would be able to lay back in bed before I had to start work. (I saw this as a perk of being able to work from home.)

I spent afternoons wishing the day would go by faster so I could finally relax with, you guessed it, a glass of wine. I was living my life one drink to the next, and it was exhausting. But the more I looked around at friends, social media, and any show on Netflix with a mom as the protagonist, the more I saw that every woman seemed to use wine as the glue holding her life together, or at least as the big reward for her stressful life.

When I decided it was time to make a change, the first essential thing I did was begin to get curious about *how* I had gotten hooked on drinking every night.

I learned we are conditioned to believe from a very young age that there are many benefits to alcohol. These beliefs are built up in our subconscious over time, meaning we aren't even aware that these beliefs are present in us.

HOW WE DEVELOPED THESE BELIEFS ABOUT ALCOHOL

Embedded within us from an early age, we're subtly conditioned to embrace the allure of alcohol, convinced of its supposed "benefits" and the societal pressure to drink it. This cultural influence weaves itself into the fabric of our subconscious, shaping our perceptions and drinking habits without us even realizing it. The journey toward freedom begins by bringing these cultural lies out of the shadows and into the light of truth.

Together, we'll delve into the manipulative tactics of big alcohol marketing, dissect the pervasive messaging of social media, reflect on the familial and peer dynamics that contribute to our beliefs, examine the portrayal of alcohol in movies and TV, and even consider how the church may have shaped the way that we think about drinking.

Big Alcohol

Like so many other women, I grew up in a world where I was conditioned from childhood to believe that alcohol held the power to make my life better: to infuse date nights with romantic allure, to make parties more fun, to offer extra relaxation on vacation, and to serve as the ultimate reward for surviving a long day with the kids. These deeply ingrained beliefs were largely shaped by the relentless marketing strategies of the largest companies in the alcohol industry, or "big alcohol."

Big alcohol doesn't just spend billions of marketing dollars each year;[1] they are maestros of narrative, crafting tales that persuade us that alcohol is the magic elixir of a happy, successful life and that we would be truly missing out if we abstained from their highly addictive products.

I recently drove by a billboard advertisement from a gin company. The photo of two people holding their drinks had one massive word written across it: *Deserved*. We are sold the idea that alcohol is a treat and a reward. Later that day, I was at a movie theater with my children, and a whiskey commercial played before the film. It showed a young man, who seemed barely over twenty-one, camping with his grandfather. They were both drinking out of matching flasks. The commercial promised connection would come with drinking their product. Next time you see an ad for alcohol, try to put your finger on what underlying promise is being sold to you. It might be belonging, success, beauty, or relaxation, all through the guise of drinking alcohol. These promises matter because they speak to us more powerfully than we think.

But it's not just big alcohol's fault that we have false beliefs about booze.

Social Media

I used to fully believe that pouring myself a glass of wine after the children had gone to bed was the be-all and end-all reward I deserved at the end of the day. And when I scrolled through Instagram, it certainly looked like other moms felt the same way. Mommy wine culture, which we will dive into later, is most pervasive on social media.

Alcohol is also the default way to celebrate anything, according to Instagram. Whether buying a new home, graduating, getting a promotion, or ringing in the new year, we're told alcohol is *the* way to commemorate it. Alcohol is inextricably linked to all holidays, due to a combination of big alcohol's marketing tactics, social norms, and family culture, and then splashed all over your friends' highlight reels.

Just take a second to think about your Instagram or TikTok feed. If it's anything like mine, you'll see memes, photos, and reels of people showcasing their drinking. Once you become aware of this stuff, it's hard to unsee it.

Family

The role that family plays in our beliefs about alcohol is different for each one of us. One of the most significant topics I cover with my clients is how their parents shaped their views of alcohol.

In my family, alcohol was part of every celebration. This was the beginning of my belief that I needed alcohol to have fun and celebrate. It took me considerable time to untangle this belief and understand that I could enjoy a party without a cocktail in my hand.

I also learned from my mother that alcohol can be a coping mechanism. In 2007, when my brother, John, got in a car accident and almost died, my mom drank to deal with the stress of his multiple operations and recovery. In 2011, my mom's dad died of suicide, and she drank to deal with the pain. When my mom passed away, I started drinking more than ever because I had learned that alcohol was a way to manage pain and cope with sadness.

Friends

When I first tried alcohol as a teenager, I thought it tasted awful. But instead of never drinking it again, I conditioned my taste buds and continued drinking through college because all my friends were doing it. I wanted to fit in. For many of us, drinking is one of the first times we experience peer pressure. It seems like the cool, hip, and mature thing to do, so most of us make ourselves "like" it.

The horrible thing about peer pressure is that it doesn't stop after high school or college. As adult women, we experience it. And I hate to admit this, but I also helped facilitate it. When a close girlfriend decided she wanted to take a month off wine, I gave her a hard time and asked her why she couldn't have just one glass. We give others a hard time for not drinking to help defend our own drinking. Sometimes it feels like we never graduated from high school, except now we find more sophisticated ways to pressure one another to indulge. "Come on, we always end the night with espresso martinis" was a favorite mantra of mine.

Entertainment

I was recently watching *Modern Family* with my children, and I noticed that Claire Dunphy, one of the main mom characters in the show, was drinking wine out of a tumbler at her son Luke's soccer game because she was overwhelmed by her current family drama. What did Olivia Pope of *Scandal* do to decompress after a long day at the office? She pulled out the red wine. What does Christina Applegate's character do in *Dead to Me* when faced with her husband's death? She drowns her sorrows in cabernet. What do the gals in *Sex and the City* do when they want to have fun? Cosmos all around.

Church

Depending on your faith community, you've possibly encountered alcohol within church. Whether it's the communion wine or alcoholic beverages served at church gatherings like picnics and barbecues or even Bible studies, the presence of alcohol in these settings can inadvertently convey some level of approval. Conversely, some of you may have been raised in church communities where alcohol was stigmatized, fostering an atmosphere of shame, blame, and negativity, thereby contributing to the perception of alcohol as a forbidden fruit. Either way, a faith community can and does play a role in shaping your thoughts and beliefs about alcohol, and it's worth considering what influence this has had on your life.

HERE'S THE GOOD NEWS

You don't have to buy into the assumption that alcohol is benefiting you. You don't have to hang on to the lie that you need alcohol to navigate life. I love *The Message* translation of today's verse. Let's look at it again: "Don't become so well-adjusted to your culture that you fit into it without even thinking. Instead, fix your attention on God. You'll be changed from the inside out. . . . Unlike the culture around you, always dragging you down . . . God brings the best out of you" (Romans 12:2).

Which cultural lie hits home for you the most? What message have you bought into without question? Is it the lie that you need alcohol to celebrate or to deal with stress? And where is that lie coming from?

I have good news for you, babe. Jesus is a better source of rest, celebration, healing, and connection than alcohol. In Him, we can find a richness of joy, fulfillment, and purpose that no amount of alcohol can ever hope to replicate.

TiNA

CONSIDER THE MEDIA YOU'VE SEEN RECENTLY THAT promotes alcohol. What underlying promises did you feel most drawn to? Connection, fun, belonging, relaxation, romance, or something else? Take out your journal and jot down what stood out to you the most about what you read today.

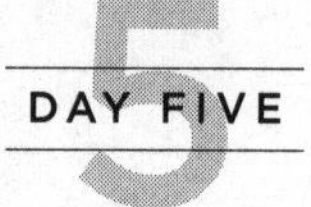

DAY FIVE

Cracking the Code

I praise you because I am fearfully and wonderfully made;
your works are wonderful,
I know that full well.

—PSALM 139:14

I USED TO FEEL LIKE I WAS THE ONLY ONE WHO COULDN'T quite crack the code when it came to drinking. Why did everyone around me seem to have this easy and carefree relationship with alcohol? They seemed to possess a hidden formula that allowed them to enjoy a drink or two without compulsion for more. Why couldn't I have that?

It seemed something was wrong with me, like I didn't have strong enough willpower. It was the same story when trying to stick to diets and exercise routines; I was never good enough. When I went on my break from alcohol, not knowing if it would be forever or not, I spent the first several months reading everything I could find about alcohol. I'll never forget the first time I read about how addictive it is. I burst into tears. I realized there wasn't anything wrong with me. God didn't skip the "able to moderate alcohol" gene when He created me. Anyone can get hooked on alcohol because of what it does to our brains and bodies. Alcohol does what alcohol does: It makes you crave another drink.

Why is that encouraging? Because it shows us that we lose the willpower battle (which we will discuss more on day ten) *not* because of who we are but because alcohol is *designed* to overrule willpower. I am not broken when it comes to alcohol, and neither are you. Alcohol got me addicted because it's addictive.

It's not up to you or me to crack the code of sticking to two drinks. It makes no sense physiologically. Here's why.

THE DOPAMINE CYCLE

When we drink, we get a temporary feeling of euphoria from the chemical hormone dopamine. The fleeting feeling only lasts about thirty minutes; after that, our dopamine levels return to baseline.[1] Dopamine is both the pleasure and learning molecule, meaning when we do something that feels good, like drinking, the brain records it as a positive experience. It cements a neural pathway that remembers, "Wine makes me feel good. Drink more wine to feel good."

For clarification, a neural pathway is like a road in your brain made of connected brain cells. These roads help you remember how to repeat an action or think a certain way.

The dose of dopamine we get from a glass of wine is unnaturally large for our system, which means our body needs to do some serious work to balance us out and bring us back to homeostasis. To do so, it releases a counter-chemical called dynorphin, a downer and sedative hormone.[2]

But the brain likes the dopamine buzz, so what do we do when we start to feel the effects of the dynorphin after about thirty minutes? We reach for another glass. This is how alcohol is highly addictive; we are constantly chasing that dopamine high.

It's important to note that this is our body's chemical reaction with all drugs. First, we get a high, and then our body counteracts the high, so we feel like we need more to maintain the buzz. Our bodies respond to alcohol in the same way they respond to drugs like cocaine and heroin. However, because alcohol is socially acceptable and we have been force-fed the narrative that it's the elixir for a good life, it's a far more pervasive issue than our culture admits.

ALCOHOL IS A DIURETIC

Think about how many glasses of juice or sparkling water you can drink in one sitting. Can you drink five or six glasses in a row? Nope. That's because those drinks satisfy your thirst, whereas alcohol dehydrates you, leaving you thirsty. Alcohol is a diuretic, simply meaning it dehydrates you.[3] You reach for the second glass immediately after you finish the first. It's why you have to chug a bottle of water in the middle of the night after drinking alcohol. You're dehydrated. In addition to chasing the dopamine high, we drink more alcohol to attempt to satisfy our thirst.

ALCOHOL HIJACKS YOUR DECISION-MAKING SYSTEM

If I had a penny for every time I broke a drinking promise to myself, I'd be a very wealthy lady. I told myself I'd stick to water between glasses, limit myself to one or two drinks, only indulge on weekends—the list goes on. But no matter how determined I was, I always ended up caving in. Why? Because alcohol messes with the two parts of our brain responsible for making choices.

The human brain is one of God's most marvelous creations. Think of your brain as having two main areas for decision-making: the prefrontal cortex (the upper brain) and the limbic system (the lower brain). The upper brain handles logical thinking, planning, self-control, and learning from mistakes.[4] On the other hand, the lower brain kicks in during emotional or threatening situations, triggering our fight-or-flight response.[5]

Alcohol tricks the lower brain into thinking that skipping a drink is a threat, hijacking our rational decision-making abilities. This confusion can lead us to make impulsive choices, like reaching for another drink even when we promised ourselves we wouldn't.

When we're well rested, hydrated, and emotionally stable, our upper brain works at its best, helping us make wise decisions. But when we're tired, stressed, or emotionally drained, the lower brain takes over, making us more susceptible to cravings and impulsive behavior.

This is why we can start our day at seven in the morning feeling confident we will not drink and by five o'clock we are pouring that first glass. By the end of the day, we are operating from our lower brain, and that end-of-the-day glass of wine suddenly feels like it's do-or-die. This is also why grace, compassion, sleep, and self-care are so important when assessing your alcohol intake. The more you can operate from the upper part of your brain, the better your chance of making a sound, non-survival-based decision.

THERE'S NOTHING WRONG WITH YOU

When I first learned all this, I was elated, then shocked, and then angry. I had been duped into believing that a highly addictive substance was supposed to help me when it actually just kept me wanting more. When the dust settled, I felt incredibly grateful to have learned I wasn't somehow defective. I was just hooked on a highly addictive substance and socially conditioned to call it normal.

Whether you already know how addictive alcohol is or are learning about this for the first time, I want you to know there is so much hope for you. God fearfully and wonderfully made you. You were knit together by God in your mother's womb.[6] Learning how your body is designed to respond to alcohol is an essential part of resetting your alcohol relationship with intentionality.

TiNA

NOW THAT YOU'RE AWARE OF THE THIRTY-MINUTE dopamine spike, take a moment to consider its impact on your past experiences. Recall a time when you were out with friends and that first glass of wine made it challenging to concentrate on the conversation because your mind was fixated on ordering the next glass. Or perhaps you can remember a time you were at home lounging on the couch and that initial glass left you yearning for a second.

Grab your journal and jot down in your own words what resonated with you the most from today's insights. Is there a sense of relief in knowing there's nothing wrong with you?

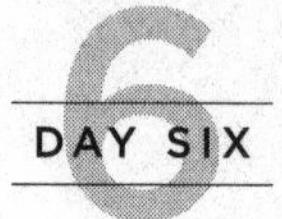

DAY SIX

The Battle in Our Brains

I do not understand what I do. For what I want to do I do not do, but what I hate I do.

—ROMANS 7:15

RECENTLY I WAS TALKING TO ONE OF MY CLIENTS, MARY, who was taking a break from wine. The first few weeks had gone smoothly. But as Thanksgiving approached and she was preparing to host her entire extended family, I could tell she was feeling less sure of her decision.

"Where is this belief coming from that Thanksgiving has to be accompanied by wine?" I asked.

She looked at me and said, "I don't know, maybe it's FOMO."

"Maybe," I replied. I thought for a second, then asked, "What were your Thanksgivings like growing up?"

She began talking about how she had watched her father drink every Thanksgiving. It had made her uncomfortable, so to numb the awkwardness, she, too, turned to wine.

We both sat back for a moment in silence; we knew we had uncovered something big. Now that Mary understood she had this subconscious belief about needing alcohol during

Thanksgiving and understood why she had this belief, she could face it, tackle it, and ask the critical question: *Is it true?* For Mary, the question went something like this: *Is it true that wine helped ease the discomfort of being with my father on Thanksgiving when he was drinking?*

Her answer was no. When Mary and her father both drank, it just caused more tension between them.

We hold thousands of beliefs in our subconscious because of how we were raised, who we hang out with, what church we went to, and what media we consume. When we pour a glass, we don't realize how our subconscious beliefs are swaying us.

Imagine your conscious mind is like a diligent librarian, meticulously organizing our beliefs as if they're individual books. Each "book" has a corresponding filing cabinet drawer in your subconscious mind. These drawers overflow with memories, experiences, and impressions supporting these beliefs. We don't always realize where our beliefs stem from—after all, the filing cabinet is old, dusty, and vast with files we've long forgotten about. But when we begin digging in that maze of subconscious files, we uncover why we think like we do—about alcohol and everything else in our lives.

For example, many women I coach think drinking gives them more confidence in social situations. I used to think I was more social when I had a few drinks. I was less anxious to chat with people I didn't know. So, how did my subconscious come up with this belief? First, while growing up, I saw alcohol served at every party my parents hosted. Then, this belief was further solidified in college at the University of Southern California. I was in a sorority, and that's what you did at parties; you drank to be social and connect. Then, after college, alcohol was involved at any party or gathering. So, the belief that I needed wine to be social was solidified. Do you share the same belief? If so, where did it begin for you?

As we embark on this fast together, our mission is to unravel the common beliefs we hold about the perceived benefits of alcohol. We'll explore whether alcohol truly aids in sleep, serves as a genuine form of self-care, or provides a reliable coping mechanism for grief. We'll also delve into the notion that we drink primarily for the taste or to ease our anxiety.

Furthermore, we'll discuss the belief that alcohol adds to our fun and brings us joy, as well as its impact on our relationships and our role as mothers. We'll even examine whether it alleviates boredom and enhances every vacation experience.

Our goal, together, is to determine where these beliefs came from. What is being stored in our own subconscious to support these beliefs? We want to figure out whether these beliefs about alcohol still serve us or hold any truth. To do this, we'll draw insights from science, the wisdom of the Bible, and our personal experiences.

In *Atomic Habits,* James Clear explains, "What you crave is not the habit itself, but the change in state it delivers. You do not crave smoking a cigarette; you crave the feeling of relief it provides. You are not motivated by brushing your teeth but rather by the feeling of a clean mouth."[1] What change in state are you looking for when you pour the glass of wine? What unmet need are you looking to meet?

Before we dive deeper, I encourage you to get curious and start uncovering your own beliefs about why you enjoy drinking. Some people may have just a few reasons, while others may have many. Today's TiNA isn't so tiny. In fact,

I've intentionally made this chapter short so you can spend some good time answering the questions below. Please do not skip this.

TiNA

WHAT ARE YOUR BELIEFS ABOUT WHY YOU LIKE TO drink?

Here are a few other helpful ways to ask the same question:

- "What is the benefit I see in drinking?"
- "What do I usually want to get out of drinking?"
- "What is the job that I am assigning to alcohol?" (This question is a client favorite.)
- "What is the unmet need I have that I am looking to wine to solve?"

Here is a list of possible answers:

I enjoy the taste of a great glass of red wine.
Alcohol gives me confidence in social settings that make me feel uncomfortable.
Drinking makes every situation more fun.
I can't fall asleep without wine.
I deserve my nightcap as a reward for working hard all day.
Drinking is romantic. I can't imagine date night without it.
Alcohol helps me cope with my stressful life.

Drinking numbs my grief and sadness.
Alcohol helps me connect with my friends and family.
Alcohol quiets my anxiety.

Now, it's your turn. Write down your answer(s) in your journal.

Remember, this is not about beating yourself up but understanding yourself better with grace and compassion. Don't worry about fixing the way you think about alcohol just yet. We'll get there, I promise. But for today, get curious about your beliefs related to alcohol and where they come from.

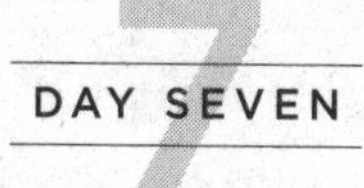

DAY SEVEN

Find Your Why

"You will seek me and find me when you seek me with all your heart. I will be found by you," declares the Lord.

—JEREMIAH 29:13–14

Unpacking our whys is essential to making a lasting change. This fast isn't just about drinking or not drinking; it's about making the most of your life while here on earth. It's about figuring out what is best for you. Yesterday, I asked you why you think you like to drink. Today, we're going to dive into a different why. *Why do you want to fast from alcohol?*

At the beginning of my alcohol reset, the reasons why I wanted to get my drinking under control poured out of me. (Pun intended.) Some of my reasons were obvious: I wanted to feel better, I didn't want to feel hungover all the time, and I wanted to get better sleep.

I also wanted to be stronger and healthier. I used to book workout classes and skip them the next morning because I didn't feel I had the energy. My body felt weak. I wasn't making healthy food choices. When I opened a wine bottle, all my plans for cooking a nutritious meal went right out the window and I would often order something unhealthy to be delivered to help me soak up all the wine.

But the biggest reason I wanted to make a change was to repair my relationships. One relationship my drinking affected was with my husband. My drinking was getting in the way of our marriage, big-time. When we both drank, we would bicker and wake up angry, not remembering what the fight was about.

If I had too much to drink and argued with Chris, before falling asleep I would try to make a note on my phone about why we argued. But of course, I still couldn't understand my drunken notes the next morning. Nothing would ever get resolved because we never remembered what we were arguing about in the first place. I felt us losing our connection and our intimacy. I felt my marriage going down the drain. I thought if I could get a handle on my drinking, things might get better.

Then there were my children. And this is *really* hard for me to write about, but I prioritized the wine over them. I used to start thinking about the wine around four o'clock on my way to school pickup. I wanted relief from the long day more than I wanted to engage with Ella and Carter. I wanted to have my own time instead of playing with them. Making their dinner and supervising their homework felt like an awful chore. When they were little, I would loathe what so many moms call "the witching hour"—dinner, bath, and bedtime. I'd rather be drinking. Reading them a bedtime story? Forget it. I'd rather have the bottle of wine open next to me on the couch while I binged episodes of *The Real Housewives of New York City*. And when I did engage with my kiddos, I had zero patience. I blame the constant low-grade irritability from being hungover. I was desperate to get through the days with them as quickly as possible so that I could sit and drink my wine. When I think back on this time, it breaks my heart. God gave me these two beautiful, wonderful children. I had prayed for them. I had begged Him to bring them to me healthy. And He had. God blessed me big-time with two wonderful kids, and I didn't even want to hang out with them because I would rather have been drinking. It makes me tear up even as I write that. Thankfully, in sobriety, I have been able to prioritize my relationships with Ella and Carter and feel closer to them than ever before.

And then, the most important relationship in my life was the one with Jesus, my Creator, my Father. I had grown so far apart from Him that I no longer recognized myself. Waking up fuzzy meant there was no time for reading my Bible in the mornings. Church on Sunday was often missed because of a wild Saturday night. I was placing so many things before my relationship with Christ. I used to pray sporadically before falling asleep, but I didn't create any space to be with God or hear from His Holy Spirit. My life felt desolate without Him.

When I think about my drinking and relationship with Jesus, I think about the prodigal son in Luke 15. To refresh your memory, Jesus told the parable of a young man who recklessly squanders his inheritance, only to find himself so hungry he's thinking about eating pig slop. When he returns home, expecting nothing but a scolding, he is instead welcomed with unconditional love and forgiveness from his father. Like this son, I had turned my back on Jesus. I ran away, taking all His blessings with me without so much as a

"Thanks, Dad." I fully immersed myself in the world, and the world gave me wine to cope with children, to reward myself, and to let my hair down. When I finally realized there is zero fulfillment in doing life this way, I returned to Jesus in tears and asked for forgiveness. And the beautiful thing is, I truly felt welcomed home by Him when I decided to make this change in my life.

So now I want to turn the question to you. Why did you pick up this book? Is it because you want to sleep better or feel better physically? Are you experiencing unbearable anxiety? Are you starting to wonder—despite the positive propaganda—if alcohol is *adding* stress to your life, not removing it? Is wine getting in the way of your ability to do your job effectively? On my coaching application form, I ask new clients, "What would be possible for you if you stopped drinking?" A woman recently wrote in response, "The world would be my oyster." Do you feel the same?

TiNA

PICK UP YOUR JOURNAL AND ANSWER TWO QUEStions:

1. Why do you want to take a break from alcohol? Write down the change you're hoping to experience.
2. What relationships would you like to improve? This may be difficult, but try to sit with any

emotion you might feel and consider how your relationship with alcohol affects your relationships with your family, your friends, and Jesus.

Keep these answers handy whenever you question your reason for doing this fast in the first place.

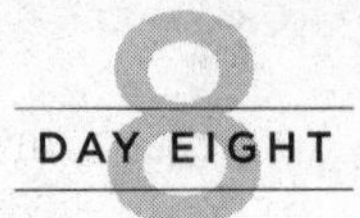

DAY EIGHT

Take Every Thought Captive

We demolish arguments and every pretension that sets itself up against the knowledge of God, and we take captive every thought to make it obedient to Christ.

—2 CORINTHIANS 10:5

WHEN WE FIRST SET OUT TO CHANGE A HABIT, WE OFTEN start by trying to modify our behavior. But where we actually need to begin is with our thoughts. Then, we need to understand further how our thoughts make us feel. Remember, we have to change our thinking to change our drinking.

One of the most life-changing realizations I had on my sobriety journey is that my relationship with alcohol isn't actually about alcohol at all. It's not about the substance. It's about my desire for how alcohol makes me *feel*. You probably picked up this book because you once liked how alcohol made you feel, but now you're not so sure. The fact that you're questioning alcohol's role in your life and exploring it is huge and should be celebrated. (If I could give you a hug and a high five right now, I would.)

CHANGING HOW WE THINK

Here's the great news: The apostle Paul gives us a road map to changing how we think. I love to think of Paul as one of the first neuroscientists because he talks so much about metacognition, a modern fancy word that means to examine your thoughts. In Romans 8:6 he said, "Letting your sinful nature control your mind leads to death. But letting the Spirit control your mind leads to life and peace" (NLT). So many clients tell me during our initial call that they feel like they have lost control over wine. To get back in the driver's seat, we must recognize how our minds have been tricked and trained to believe that alcohol is somehow benefiting us. As Paul wrote to the Corinthians in today's verse, we must take every thought (including thoughts about alcohol) captive.

Because (and I want you to remember this) when we change our thoughts, we can change the way we feel, and then we are equipped to change our behaviors.

Our thoughts can be hard to change, so how do we do this work effectively and with grace? Here's how I like to think about it:

AWARENESS → STORY → TRUTH

Let's break this out into small steps.

Step One: Become Aware of the Thought

You're already a step ahead here. You did this on day six when you listed *why* you like to drink. It may not seem like a huge deal, but when you made that list, you took a careful look at the experiences and assumptions that have determined your beliefs about alcohol.

Your brain has had a lifetime to collect data to support your beliefs, and it may take some time for you to become fully aware of all these subconscious thoughts. The second we bring these thoughts and beliefs into the light, we can decide if they still hold any merit.

Step Two: Investigate the Story

Our minds are meaning-making machines, constantly writing stories based on all the data they receive from the world. In his book, *Healing What You Can't Erase,* Christopher Cook writes, "We human beings are wired for story, and we all write them inside the recesses of our minds. Our brains are hardwired to string memories together in narrative form to construct meaning from our life experiences. The stories we tell ourselves form our expectations and hope—our outlook on life."[1]

Sometimes the stories are true, and sometimes they are pure fiction. Let's say I'm supposed to meet a girlfriend for dinner at seven o'clock, and at six forty-five, after my babysitter has walked in my front door, I get a text from my friend that reads, "So sorry. Have to cancel." Immediately I think how rude and inconsiderate my friend is. *She knew I had a babysitter coming. What a flake.* But the truth is I have no idea what's going on with my friend. Maybe her child is sick, or maybe there's been an emergency. Instead of taking the text for what it is, I've created a massive story around it. My brain has filled in the gaps with things that may not be true.

Each story our thoughts create can be separated into two

parts: the story and the facts. Take the text message example. The *facts* are that my friend could no longer attend dinner. The *story* was all the meaning I attached to the situation.

We do the same with drinking. Our minds create stories about why we like and "need" alcohol. Without careful examination (taking the thought captive), we believe these stories are true.

For example, I believed alcohol was helping my sleep. The *fact* was that it made me pass out, but I had created a *story* that it was helping me rest. I had to investigate whether or not that story was true by doing my own research and testing it out (i.e., trying to sleep without wine). Which brings us to our next step.

Step Three: What's the Truth?

Now that we know some of our beliefs about alcohol might not be actual facts, we can figure out the truth. And here again, you're already a step ahead. Much of figuring out the truth is in testing our beliefs in real life, which we're doing now with this forty-day fast.

My thoughts and beliefs about alcohol and sleep changed immediately once I learned the truth about how it hijacks my sleep (which we'll cover more on day sixteen) and once I got proper rest without drinking wine.

When I began my break from alcohol, I knew the story that would be the hardest to investigate was that alcohol equaled fun. I had to go out and do things—go to parties, meet up with friends, go on vacations, and experience holidays *without* alcohol to test if I would have zero fun without it. Good news again: When I tested that belief by removing alcohol from social events, I discovered that life without alcohol is much more fun than life with it. If that feels like a totally impossible thought for you right now, that's okay. Trust the process of God renewing your mind. His timing is perfect.

GOD'S TRUTH

If we don't run our thoughts and stories through God's truth, they will run our lives and cause us to show up as people we don't want to be. We need truth. In John 8:32, Jesus says that knowing His truth, His gospel, will set us free. Hebrews 4:12 says, "For the word of God is living and active, sharper than any two-edged sword, piercing to the division of soul and of spirit, of joints and of marrow, and discerning the thoughts and intentions of the heart" (ESV). One of the best things about being a Christian is that we have access to truth in the Bible.

Many of the women I coach drink because of stress and anxiety. When we dive deep into the stories they subconsciously created, the root of the story is often about their worth. They want to do better, be better, be thinner, be a better mother, have it all, and be it all for their families and friends. It all becomes too much, and they want to shut off the constant pressure of trying to live up to unrealistic versions of themselves. The easy-button answer is alcohol. These thoughts that negate our worth are the thoughts we need to take captive and run through the filter of what God says about us.

You are loved and worthy of God's love even if you didn't get everything checked off on your to-do list. Even if your kids didn't make the team or get into that school. Even if you were skipped over for that promotion or if you messed up that project, your true worth is unchanged. God loves you so much that He sent His Son to the cross. So, if you're drinking because you feel you're not enough, the truth is you're God's daughter. Meditating on that truth can change your behavior. When you fully comprehend that God sees you as worthy, that He knows and loves you, the pressure is off and so is the need to numb with alcohol.

You can use this truth-finding tactic for everything in your life, not just as it relates to your drinking. Anytime you feel pressure or discomfort, take a minute to observe your thoughts, figure out what story your brain might be making up, and check it against God's truth.

TiNA

TRY OUT THIS EXERCISE TODAY. REMEMBER A RECENT time you felt angry, upset, sad, disappointed, or annoyed. In your journal, reflect on these questions:

1. What thoughts occurred to you in response to that emotion?
2. What was the story you were telling yourself? Separate the story from the facts.
3. How might you rewrite the story to be more truthful?
4. How has incorporating God's truth shifted the emotion?

DAY NINE

Ditching the Label

> *See how very much our Father loves us, for he calls us his children, and that is what we are!*
>
> —1 JOHN 3:1, NLT

After I graduated from college, I went on a celebratory trip to Mexico with a few girlfriends. One moment from this trip stands out in my memory. My friend and I were sitting by the pool one day, drinking margaritas, and I told her, "Being an alcoholic would be the absolute worst thing in the world. Imagine being told you could never drink. Especially in a place like this."

Many years later, I sat in my London home in the middle of the night googling, "Am I an alcoholic?" Every time I googled this question, I always found a reason why my drinking didn't merit that label. After all, my hands never shook from withdrawals. I never drank before lunch, except at a weekend brunch, of course. It was confusing to me because as I looked at friends around me and as I scrolled through social media, no one seemed to be drinking differently than I was. If they didn't have a problem, maybe I didn't either?

But a big part of me knew alcohol was getting in the way.

I was starting to see what it was costing me. I thought alcoholics were dysfunctional people who drank whiskey out of brown paper bags on park benches. I was a mom with two great kids; I was the brand manager for a popular wellness platform; I traveled around Europe on press trips so I could write a blog for expats. Surely, I didn't qualify for the label. But as I began my own fast, I realized one reason I was stuck in my drinking was because I was petrified of the stigma attached to the label "alcoholic."

If you've gone down the Google rabbit hole like I have, you will know there are dozens of tests to gauge whether or not one is an alcoholic. Some of them focus on the actual number of drinks or units. One test I found asked me to figure out how many units I was drinking per week, and if I was under a certain amount, I was off the hook. Certainly, if I could go a few nights here and there drinking zero units, then I didn't have "a problem."

This might sound controversial, but there isn't a diagnostic DNA test that can confirm whether you're an alcoholic or not. Otherwise, we'd be able to get our answer right there on 23andMe. The reality is more nuanced. According to an in-depth study published in *Nature Neuroscience,* addiction arises from a complex interplay of multiple genes, not just one solitary culprit.[1] Another large-scale study by the National Institute on Alcohol Abuse and Alcoholism (NIAAA) tells us that it's not just about a set of genes but how those genes are affected by our environment that influences a person's likelihood of getting hooked on booze.[2]

So yes, genes are something to consider, but they aren't the definitive cause.

If you go to the doctor and say, "I think I might be drinking too much," they may ask you a set of questions and then decide, using their subjective judgment, whether your answers warrant giving you the label of "alcoholic" (although now, the medical community is moving away from using the term). I've coached women who have told their doctor that they are drinking most nights and the doctor's response is, "Seems fine to me." Their drinking then continued at the same rate because of one individual who—though medically trained—didn't fully grasp how alcohol was negatively affecting their mental health, relationships, and day-to-day life.

Even though the label makes little sense, we fear the stigma. There are "alcoholics," and then there are "normal drinkers," and we are desperate to be normal. We are so scared that this word means something is wrong with *us* that we justify our behavior like I did during all that late-night googling.

If the label helps and empowers you, by all means, use it. But the ruling of whether a subjective label does or does not apply shouldn't get in the way of you living your best life for the good of others and the glory of God. Remember, there isn't anything wrong with you: Alcohol is the problem because it's extremely addictive. My client Allison said, "The label doesn't serve me because it made me feel so weak and at fault. Removing the label and understanding that the fault is with alcohol and *not me* was life-changing!"

No one, including *you,* has to use any sort of label if you don't want to. I personally don't use the label "alcoholic," and I don't refer to myself as having a "drinking problem." The labels don't empower me. Some women I've coached don't like the word "sober," so I suggest they avoid it.

If any labels are holding you back, give yourself permission to leave them behind.

BETTER QUESTIONS AND BETTER LABELS

Instead of wondering whether you're an alcoholic or not, try asking these better questions:

"Would I have more energy if I wasn't drinking?"
"Would I sleep better without a glass of wine tonight?"
"Would I stop getting into so many stupid fights with my husband if I wasn't buzzed all the time?"
"Would I have more patience and kindness for my family if I wasn't hungover this weekend?"
"Would not drinking lower my overall anxiety?"

If you said yes to any of the questions above, taking a break from booze is so worthwhile to give yourself the chance to reset and determine if it's genuinely still serving you.

Instead of "alcoholic," let's find some truer labels to focus on. The Bible refers to us as God's children over twenty-five times! Here are some of my other favorite identities that I choose to cling to:

God's beloved child (Ephesians 5:1)
A new creation in Him (2 Corinthians 5:17)
Ambassador for Christ (2 Corinthians 5:20)
Citizen of heaven (Philippians 3:20)
Salt of the earth and the light of the world (Matthew 5:13–14)
Chosen by God (John 15:16)

Those are labels that help and empower us. These are the names we can lean into, the ones that God gives us.

TiNA

RETURN TO THE LIST OF BIBLICAL IDENTITIES AND pick one or two that resonate with you the most.

The next time you sense the urge to pour a glass, think about the name God has given you as a reminder of who you really are.

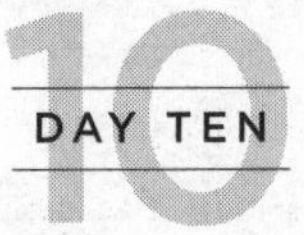

DAY TEN

The Willpower Trap

Jesus looked at them and said, "With man this is impossible, but with God all things are possible."

—MATTHEW 19:26

BEFORE I QUIT DRINKING FOR GOOD, I TRIED THE DRY January challenge several times. I remember the first year being completely miserable. At the time, I was working in a job that I really didn't enjoy, running the public relations and business development departments for a London-based start-up. I would come home exhausted to two little kids, and all I wanted to do was open up a bottle of red wine. But I knew I needed a break from booze, so I white-knuckled my way through each evening.

On January 29, I closed a big account at work and ordered a bottle of wine at dinner with a girlfriend. "I deserve this!" I said. I had relied on willpower the whole month. I had done no work on my thoughts or beliefs behind my drinking. So opening the wine bottle was automatic when that need for a reward popped up. My willpower was utterly depleted.

The following year, I decided to try Dry January again. It had been a particularly boozy December (which includes my birthday, my wedding anniversary, and Christmas), and I knew I needed a break. I approached Dry January as punishment for too much cocktailing. This time my willpower did see me through the full thirty-one days. But you know what happened on February 1? The wheels came off. In the weeks following I wound up drinking even more than I had drunk in December. It was like Dry January never even happened. My habits and thoughts hadn't changed. In fact, those beliefs were compounded with new evidence that if I could go thirty-one days without alcohol, it meant I didn't have a "problem" and could continue drinking like I had been. If I could make it a month, I had no issue.

Through both challenges, I was miserable the entire time. Using willpower alone without doing any other work made me feel deprived, just like in dieting. It made me feel like I was missing out. Willpower means consciously and deliberately making decisions to resist temptations and cravings, even if it goes against your subconscious desire. It means saying no to something your subconscious brain really wants. But if you reevaluate the desire (the reasons you like to drink that you identified on day six), then you don't need to rely on willpower in the first place.

Your conscious mind might tell you, "This wine is just going to make me feel crummy in the morning," but your subconscious mind believes the alcohol is helping you relax. When you rely on willpower, you ignore all the data from your subconscious, which has built up underlying beliefs over decades. It's like when I opened the bottle of wine on January 29 after closing the account at work. My subconscious belief that wine was a reward overruled my willpower not to drink. I could not strong-arm or overcome a deeply held belief by fleeting willpower. Do you see how, again, it all starts in our minds? Change your thinking, change your drinking.

Most people believe willpower is like a muscle, and the more you work it, the stronger it gets, but that's a misconception. Willpower is more like a battery that slowly loses power throughout the day. It can only carry you so far. You have a set amount of willpower when you wake up in the morning. Decisions come at you hard and fast from the moment you open your eyes. Sure, most of these decisions don't have to do with your drinking, but your brain is in decision-making mode all day long. By evening, when the choice is, "Shall I have just one glass?" you've got what's known as "decision fatigue." Your willpower battery is dead, and you cave and have a glass of wine.

You'll be glad to know that you and I aren't alone in the willpower struggle. Let's look a little more closely at a verse from earlier. Paul wrote, "I do not understand what I do. For what I want to do I do not do, but what I hate I do. . . . For I do not do the good I want to do, but the evil I do not want to do—this I keep on doing" (Romans 7:15, 19). Paul fully recognized that on his own, he couldn't strong-arm his brain into doing certain actions that he wanted to do. He had to go deeper. Paul knew the way to change our behavior starts in our minds. It starts with taking every thought captive and then figuring out what part is story and what part is truth.

Can I tell you the *really* good news? When you combine this work in your subconscious with prayer, true and lasting transformation happens! When you ask God to reveal what you believe is the benefit of wine, He helps you uncover the truth. Ephesians 3:20 says, "Now to him who is able to do far more abundantly than all that we ask or think, according to the power at work within us" (ESV). When we ask for God's help, He can unlock and show us things that can, in my experience, be life-changing.

TiNA

TAKE SOME TIME TODAY TO THINK BACK ON ALL THE times you've tried to take a break from alcohol. It's time to head to our journal again and consider these questions as they relate to previous alcohol fasts you've attempted or completed: Did you rely on willpower alone? How did it feel? Did it change your drinking in the long run? How do you want this time to be different?

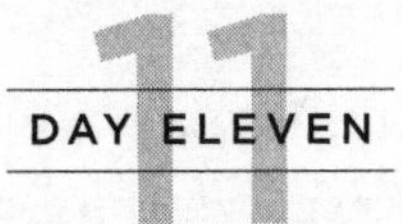

DAY ELEVEN

Prime with Prayer

Don't fret or worry. Instead of worrying, pray. Let petitions and praises shape your worries into prayers, letting God know your concerns. Before you know it, a sense of God's wholeness, everything coming together for good, will come and settle you down.

—PHILIPPIANS 4:6–7, MSG

BEFORE I STOPPED DRINKING, MY PRAYER LIFE LOOKED like this: a few words before meals with the kids, a laundry list of things I was worried about right after my head hit the pillow, and pleading for a good parking spot when I was late for Pilates. (Full disclosure: I *still* pray for that parking spot.) And then there were the prayers about my drinking, which were often muttered as I was about to fall asleep, *God, I know I shouldn't be drinking like this*. I also remember praying, *I know You see me,* and hoping He would send some divine rescue team.

But I never told God I wanted to stop drinking. I wasn't ready. Deep down, I still believed wine was the glue holding everything together. I still believed it was my ultimate reward for being a hardworking mom. But after I stopped drinking, my prayer life radically changed. When I started sleeping properly, my body naturally woke up around five in the morning when the house was quiet and everyone was still sleeping. So I started getting up early. I would make coffee, sit on the couch with Copper, my cavapoo, and pray. I prayed a lot of teary prayers in those first months. I cried over 2 Corinthians 12:9–10, which reminded me that God's power is made perfect in my weakness. And through my prayer time, I began to feel closer to Jesus than I had in decades.

I used to hear women at Bible study say, "God spoke to me and said . . ." and I wondered, *How do they do that? Why is God speaking to them and not to me?* But in sobriety, I learned that I hadn't made space for God to speak to me. I wasn't regularly in the Word. Psalm 46:10 says, "Be still, and know that I am God," but I never got still. How could I hear Him or try to understand His purpose for me if I never got still? If I never got quiet? The wine turned off my ability to hear from God. My constant buzz was drowning out His voice.

Those early five o'clock quiet times made it possible.

During those mornings, I began practicing gratitude and acknowledging and thanking Him for my numerous blessings—something I never stopped to do when I was drinking. I brought my requests before the Lord in a new way. I learned that prayer was a two-way street because if I held space for Jesus, His Holy Spirit would talk right back, just like He did for the women in Bible study.

I realized that when I opened the Bible and started reading it and praying over it, I could hear the Lord's voice loud and clear, guiding, directing, comforting, and telling me that He had a strong purpose for me. And I realized He had been there all along, even through my disordered drinking battle, even if I wasn't making space for Him.

When was the last time you stopped to hold space for

Jesus and hear from Him? Listen, I know it's always hard to make time. I bet you're super busy, just like me, and when you read the words "five o'clock in the morning," you think it's unrealistic. But let me remind you that prayer is the most important thing you can do in your whole day.

When I am too rushed during the day to squeeze in time with Jesus, I feel the consequences. I am more anxious. I start to rely on my own ability, as opposed to putting my total trust in Him. I get caught up in the little things instead of focusing on what really matters.

I find this time most regularly in the early morning, but it doesn't have to be early for you. Find the time that works best for you: after you drop the kids at school, on your lunch break, or in your car while you commute. Putting on worship music and praying in the car has also been a total game changer for me. There's nothing like a little Maverick City Music when sitting in traffic to bring me peace and calm in the chaos.

I remember one morning in rush hour blasting the song "Promises."[1] When I looked up, God had placed a rainbow right there for me as I sang and prayed in the car. If I had been hungover, I would never have had that connection with God. Making space for prayer—not just to talk at Jesus, but to listen to what He has to say to you—will help you, too, fall in love with your life again.

PRIME YOUR DAY

Mark Batterson wrote about starting our days with prayer in *The Circle Maker*. "Prayer is priming. Prayer puts us in a spiritual frame of mind. Prayer helps us see and seize the God-ordained opportunities that are all around us all the time."[2] He explains how two Dutch researchers experimented with a group of students, asking them forty-two questions from Trivial Pursuit. However, they were split into two groups before they got to the game. Group one was told to sit and think about what it meant to become a university professor; the other group was told to think about soccer. The professor group got 55.6 percent of the questions right, but the soccer group only got 42.5 percent correct. The point Batterson made is that the professor group was in the right state of mind to win the game, but the soccer group wasn't.[3] When we start our day with Jesus, we're in the right mind frame to allow Him to guide us throughout our day.

Your days will be primed one way or another. But the invitation is open to you: Start your day with Jesus.

TiNA

PRIME YOUR DAY. IDENTIFY WHAT MIGHT BE THE BEST time to make space in your day for Jesus. It might take a few tries to find a consistent rhythm, but even a handful of minutes will make a big difference. If you feel, like I did, that this break from alcohol is a struggle, bring your honest thoughts and worries to Him and let Him remind you that He is doing incredible things in your journey.

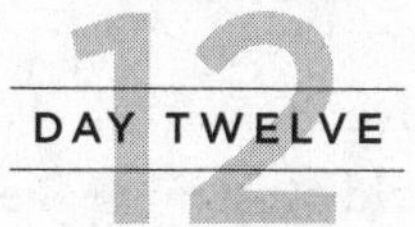

Understanding Triggers and Habits

For our light and momentary troubles are achieving for us an eternal glory that far outweighs them all.

—2 CORINTHIANS 4:17

ABOUT TEN MONTHS AFTER I QUIT ALCOHOL, I HAD NO desire to drink it anymore. I knew I would never go back to the way I was before. I did a lot of mindset work, stayed committed to uncovering my unconscious beliefs, and leaned into God. With my focus and His direction, I was on a new path. But one December day, I got a phone call that devastated me beyond words. One of my dearest girlfriends had died. She left a loving husband and three beautiful daughters behind. And the first thing I thought was, *I could use a drink*.

I've shared before how I used alcohol to numb the pain of losing my mother, and this all-too-familiar feeling brought up the same thought pattern in my head. My brain started spinning those same stories about how sauvignon blanc would somehow help me deal with the fact that my sweet friend was gone. At first, I was stunned and confused by those returning thoughts. But I took them captive and recognized them as a false narrative. The truth was, alcohol would not help me grieve. It would only make me more depressed.

Looking back, I can see that my friend's death was a massive emotional trigger for me. But because I recognized it for what it was, I could stand firm. Understanding triggers is key to changing our drinking.

WHAT ARE TRIGGERS?

A trigger can be any kind of stimulus that elicits a reaction.[1] Let's take a look at four common types of triggers.[2]

An *emotional trigger* is a specific feeling that makes you want to drink. For example, you feel lonely and reach for a bottle of wine to escape this feeling. My big emotional trigger was grief; when I felt sad, I only knew how to manage this feeling by drinking.

Environmental triggers are places or environments that elicit the impulse to drink, like the pool, your favorite restaurant, concerts, or the bar by your office. My client Melissa told me she always felt the urge to drink when she lounged on her sunny back patio.

Then, there are *exposure triggers*. These are when someone offers you a drink or there is alcohol at the party you're at or you stumble upon the wine aisle at the grocery store.

Lastly, *temporal triggers* are tied to dates and holidays—the Fourth of July, your birthday, and Christmas. For example, a client told me Saturdays were a trigger because she had spent every Saturday drinking for as long as she could remember.

Triggers can seem overwhelming—especially if we face them multiple times a day—but knowing how to respond from conscious choice, not out of subconscious impulse, is key to overcoming them.

HOW HABITS ARE FORMED

Every time that you experience one of these triggers and then have a drink, your brain forms a new neural pathway in your beautiful God-created brain. And every time you repeat the action, the link between the trigger and drinking becomes stronger. This is how we develop habits. It takes time to untie this link. It may be hard to even recognize the trigger because you're so used to the habit. My daily trigger was at five in the evening when the kids got home from school. I reached for the bottle of wine without even acknowledging it was a response to a trigger. Can you relate?

Identifying your triggers enables you to respond to stimuli with intentional choice, not habit. I found one of the best ways to interrupt my habit loop was by making a mocktail. Every afternoon after I was done with work and the kids were done with their schooling, I poured ginger ale into a crystal tumbler and added a splash of cranberry and fresh lime. My son, nine at the time, called it a "pink lady," and the kids got in on the action, requesting pink ladies each evening. Mocktail making can be a great way to begin rebuilding that trigger-habit neural pathway.

When you experience a trigger, try replacing drinking with one of these alternative actions:

Go for a walk
Meditate on your favorite Bible verse

Write down a list of things that you are thankful for
Go back to your list of whys you made on day seven
Make a list of all the positive benefits you've experienced so far when you've chosen not to drink (better sleep, more energy, etc.)
Put on your favorite song
Take a bath
Write in your journal
Make a mocktail
Say a prayer
Call a friend

As Psalm 138:3 promises, God hears and answers your prayers. He will give you strength.

MAKING HABITS STICK

When building any new habit, the key to making it stick is this: *The new habit has to feel good.* The ultimate reason I never want to go back to booze is that it feels better living without it. I am less anxious. I sleep better. I am a better mother, which feels *so* good. I have more time. My marriage is stronger. It may take some time to feel better as your brain and body heal, but stick with this.

I want to encourage you today—if you're finding it tricky to say no to alcohol because you're feeling deprived, focus on what you are *gaining* through this journey. I promise what you're gaining is so much more than what you're losing.

A NOTE ON SUMMER

Having coached many women through the seasons, it's important to give summer a special mention because of its numerous potential triggers. Vacation mode brings up the emotional triggers of wanting rest or fun, outdoor spaces like the beach or the patio are often automatically linked to cocktails, and the exposure triggers are in full effect.

My client Emily started working with me at Christmastime and was worried about the holiday season and the triggers it would bring with it. Still, when summertime rolled around she declared that, even with months of sobriety under her belt and a few helpful growth points along the way, summer was the more challenging time for her based on the number of triggers she was faced with all at once. Don't be discouraged if you're starting this fast in the summer. It may be difficult, but we can do hard things with Christ, and this time period will offer you lots of opportunities to learn about yourself and the stories you believe when it comes to alcohol.

Remember that practice makes perfect and each time you do something sober that you'd normally do while drinking, you're breaking that habit loop and reinforcing a new, healthier neural pathway.

A NOTE ON ALCOHOL-FREE SUBSTITUTES

For the majority of the women I have coached, having an alcohol-free alternative has proven helpful when interrupting drinking patterns. However, there are women who may find that having an alcohol-free wine, beer, or spirit falls into the exposure-trigger category. Don't be nervous about this; just experiment. If swapping out your nightly Corona with a Corona Non-Alcoholic (they taste exactly the same) works for you—great. If having the alcohol-free beer makes you desperate for the real thing, try something else. This is about curiosity. You won't know until you try. And don't forget, using a pretty glass is a big part of the ritual.

TiNA

GET OUT YOUR JOURNAL. TAKE A FEW MINUTES to reflect on when you most feel the impulse to drink. Then, for each of the four categories (emotional, environmental, exposure, and temporal), write down the triggers you experience.

Now, go back through the list, and alongside each trigger, write down something you can do instead of drinking. For example, if I am experiencing an exposure trigger of being offered a drink, I will ask for ginger ale. If I am experiencing an emotional trigger of loneliness, I will call my best friend. Next, circle the triggers you cannot avoid (such as a sunny day or when the kids come home from school) just as a way of flagging the ones that might be tricky to avoid.

I've done an example for you here.

CATEGORY	TRIGGER	NEW ACTION
1. *Emotional*	Feelings of grief	Open my Bible.
	Feeling lonely	Call my best friend or schedule a date night.
2. *Environmental*	Arrive at the beach with the kids for spring break	When I'm at the beach, I'll open a great beach read or go for a walk.
3. *Exposure*	Walk into a party, offered a cocktail	When I'm offered a drink at a party, I'll ask for a Diet Coke.
4. *Temporal*	Christmas party season	I'll stock up on nonalcoholic sparkling champagne to bring to celebrations and serve at home.

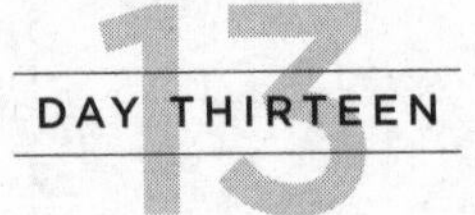

DAY THIRTEEN

Overcome the Urge to Drink

No temptation has overtaken you except what is common to mankind. And God is faithful; he will not let you be tempted beyond what you can bear. But when you are tempted, he will also provide a way out so that you can endure it.

—1 CORINTHIANS 10:13

MY CLIENT LINDSAY WAS EIGHT MONTHS INTO HER alcohol-free journey. She was preparing to travel for a work trip and was considering trying a glass of wine to determine whether the allure she had associated with it was still there. She wanted to see if it would still bring her relaxation and ease social anxiety. Because I knew Lindsay's story well, I suggested a strategic growth point to test it out. Remember, a growth point is the decision to have a drink during a period of abstinence. These can be highly effective to learn additional truths about how alcohol is genuinely making you feel, especially when you plan ahead and make a conscious decision surrounding what "benefit" you specifically want to challenge. Having a specifically trained sobriety coach can really help with these.

Lindsay conducted her growth point like a pro. She made

the conscious decision to drink a glass of red wine. One led to three, and she took notes during her experience. She wrote about how her face flushed and her hands became numb. Her verdict—"I would rank the experience of drinking that wine somewhere between neutral and unpleasant"—was that the temporary buzz wasn't that great. Lindsay had truly believed that wine felt good until she conducted that growth point and experienced what alcohol was doing to her neurochemically.

Before we dive into some of my favorite coaching tactics, I want to take a second to acknowledge the fact that alcohol does, of course, offer a buzz—a temporary feeling of euphoria. If it didn't, none of us would have gotten hooked in the first place. But be open to the idea that the feeling might not be as satisfying as we've been conditioned to believe it is.

Taking a break from alcohol is like conducting a benefit comparison analysis. In one column titled "the benefits of drinking," you could list that you have a brief buzz; in the other, "the benefits of not drinking," you have a laundry list of benefits—like better sleep, health, mental clarity, and so much more. *You* get to decide if it's worth it.

Let's dive into some practical tactics for how to handle cravings.

TACTIC I: HALT

Take a minute and figure out what your craving thoughts are telling you. Another way of asking this question: What is the unmet need that your brain has learned a drink would help with? Are you **H**ungry, **A**ngry, **L**onely, or **T**ired?[1] Our goal now is to find a way to fill that need with something that will help us, for real, and not make us feel worse.

Hungry: If you're hungry, try eating a snack or meal, ensuring that you have protein and fat to help your blood sugar balance.

Angry: If you're angry about something, take a second to pray and ask for God's peace.

Lonely: Community is also super important when you're on this journey. Reach out to a friend who might be interested in doing this fast alongside you. Find a sobriety coach or get plugged into a small coaching group. I run regular intimate coaching groups of women, and I'd love to have you join us. (See the resources section on page 225.) Boredom also may come into play here, but we will spend a whole day on that job on day thirty-two.

Tired: I hear you, sister. But alcohol hijacks sleep, so drinking is just going to make you more tired the next morning. If you're exhausted, lie down and take a nap. Or try going to bed earlier. The less you drink, the more your body will be able to get proper healing and restorative rest. Play the long game here.

TACTIC 2: PLAY THE TAPE FORWARD TWICE

This is one of my clients' favorite tactics because it's simple, easy, and helpful for overcoming a craving. It's all about visualizing how the next twenty-four hours will look if you choose to drink now. For example, this is what my tape would look like on a typical night at home.

Promise myself I will only have one glass of wine.
End up drinking more than I wanted to.
Stay up later than I should.
Pass out.
Wake up at three in the morning feeling awful, wishing I could have kept that promise to myself to have the one glass.
Finally fall asleep just before my alarm goes off to get the kids up for school.
Have a raging headache, snap at the children, be short-tempered with my whole family.
Miss my already-paid-for scheduled workout session.
Do my best to finish the day, counting the hours until bedtime.
Start making the "I'm not going to drink tonight" promises again . . .
Open the wine bottle.
Repeat.

Then, I would play the tape forward as if I hadn't had a drink. That tape would look something like this.

Read or watch television for a bit after the kids go to bed.
Get a good night's rest (not waking up at three o'clock).
Wake up, feel rested, maybe read my Bible before everyone is awake.
Move my body because it feels good, not because I am punishing myself for drinking.

Approach the day's work with a clear head and zero hangover-induced anxiety ("hangxiety").
Feel excited to pick up the kids from school and hear about their day.

When I play both tapes forward, it's a no-brainer. Why would I choose the drinking tape over the not-drinking tape? For thirty minutes of euphoria? No thanks.

TACTIC 3: THE WINE WITCH

My craving voice always sounded the same: "Just have one glass. You'll be able to moderate this time. You deserve it; it's been a long day. You have enough time to sleep it off tomorrow." We learned in earlier chapters that this voice comes from your lower brain, and it's convinced alcohol is necessary for survival because of the way we've wired that neural pathway. This isn't the logical and calm tone of your true inner voice. This is the voice of the craving. In other words, the craving voice isn't *you,* and you aren't the craving. The craving voice is impulsive and emotional, like a toddler throwing a fit because they're not getting what they want. You have the ability to take the craving thoughts captive.

It helped me to see this voice as separate from my actual voice. Clare Pooley, who wrote *The Sober Diaries,* calls her inner drinking voice a "wine witch."[2] I love that idea, but you can name your voice whatever you want.

Here are the important parts of this tactic. When you hear the voice:

- Recognize the voice as a neural pathway that has been built up over time.
- Notice that she has a one-track mind: to get you to drink.
- Remember, *you* are stronger than her.

Sometimes I like to think of this voice as a witch, and sometimes I think of her as a toddler wanting ice cream. What happens when one of your children demands ice cream and you say no? They nag you and nag you and nag you. "But pleeeeeeaseeeeee, Mommmmy!" They want the dopamine hit from the sugar like you do when you want wine. You're the boss though. You're in charge here. You get to make a conscious choice and can say, "No thanks!"

TACTIC 4: SURF THE URGE

Cravings feel like they will last forever, but they don't. They don't last nearly as long as we expect them to. When we resist cravings, we experience temporary discomfort but ultimately greater satisfaction after we've surfed the urge. When the craving begins, pick up your phone and turn on your timer for fifteen minutes. While you wait, say a prayer, pick up the Bible, or write down a few things you're grateful for. See how you are feeling after fifteen minutes. Notice whether the craving is still there or has subsided. Pay close attention to how it feels in your body and how it dissipates.

I recently had the privilege of coaching a client named Stephanie, who sent me a text amid the throes of an exceptionally intense craving. When we reconvened for our next coaching session, I asked, "How long did that craving feel like it lasted?"

She met my gaze and replied, "It felt like an eternity."

I pressed further, "And now, with the benefit of hindsight, how long would you say it actually lasted?"

Stephanie pondered momentarily and said, "Probably fifteen or twenty minutes." A shared smile between us spoke volumes.

TACTIC 5: PERSEVERANCE AND STRENGTH IN CHRIST JESUS

Overcoming a craving can feel like we are in the heat of battle, and this is the opportune time to lean into what God says about difficulties. The Bible tells us that we can do all things through Christ, who strengthens us.[3] That's right, we can do *all things*. Including dealing with intense cravings for alcohol. What God promised to Paul in 2 Corinthians 12:9 is His promise to us too: "My grace is sufficient for you, for my power is made perfect in weakness." So, even though you may feel weak when you're experiencing a craving, God is creating something so mighty in you. It may be hard to see now, but it's happening.

When a craving comes, meditate on His truth. It can help to have a notebook of your favorite Bible passages handy. Open it up and read the verses. Pray over them. Get still and ask God to sit with you in the craving and help you overcome it. Pray for the unmet need you are longing for, whether it's rest, relief, or connection. Ask God how He can help you fill that need.

TiNA

TAKE OUT YOUR JOURNAL AND PLAY THE TAPE FORWARD. Write down in detail what your night and next day would look like if you had a drink. Then, write down what happens if you don't have the drink. Pay particular attention to how you will feel in both scenarios. Flag this journal entry to refer back to when the next craving comes.

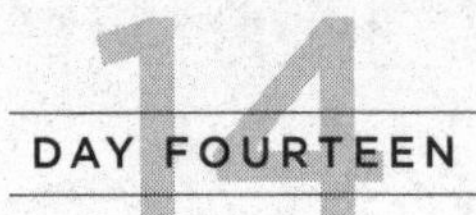

DAY FOURTEEN

Navigating Sugar Cravings

If you find honey, eat just enough—
too much of it, and you will vomit.

—PROVERBS 25:16

ONE MORNING, I WOKE UP TO A MESSAGE FROM A CLIENT with a photo attached of a massive pile of candy. Gummy bears, Sour Patch Kids, Twix, Snickers, you name it. The message said, "What do I do about these sugar cravings?!"

It's one of the most frequent questions I get from clients, and I always start with the good news that this part of the journey doesn't last forever. As I told my client in my response to her message, the two important things to remember are grace and self-compassion. When I began my alcohol-free journey, I massively craved sugar. At the end of the day, I would typically have a scoop of ice cream or several pieces of chocolate. My body was desperate for sugar, and there's a reason for that.

It's common to think that we crave sugar because our bodies are used to the sugar in alcohol, and that is partially true. However, when we reach for the candy, our body isn't looking for sugar as much as it craves the same dopamine hit we get from a drink. Remember, dopamine is the pleasure molecule, and it's also a learning molecule. Our bodies are still traveling the neural pathway we created: It's five o'clock, so it's time for a dopamine rush. And sugar is an alternative for getting that dopamine release.

Here's why I am big on grace and compassion with ourselves when it comes to the early days of sobriety. If you want to take a break from alcohol successfully, it's essential to concentrate on one thing at a time. Many of my clients start to feel so much better after giving up alcohol that they immediately want to do an entire diet overhaul and start training for a marathon. *(I'm kidding. Kind of.)* As I mentioned earlier, studies show that people who tried to accomplish multiple goals were less committed and less likely to succeed than those who focused on a single goal.[1] Our goal with this forty-day fast is to figure out if you feel better without alcohol in your day-to-day life. So focus on that, and don't beat yourself up for eating a little ice cream or having a little extra chocolate.

It also helps to not think of sugar as the enemy. We will never be able to eliminate sugar altogether from our diets. Natural forms of sugar are present in fruits and vegetables and are a source of energy. Of course, sugar is not great for our diet in highly processed forms like cookies and candy bars. But when it comes to nutrient-dense whole foods like fruit, it *can* have a place in our diet. While alcohol is a substance we can eliminate 100 percent from our diets, we can't do the same with sugar. We have to make peace with that.

Let's look at how we can use nutrition to help get our sugar cravings under control.

BALANCE YOUR BLOOD SUGAR

Sugar bombs like cookies and candy are a fast-burning energy source, but if we put more protein, healthy fat, and complex carbohydrates into our diets in thoughtful ways, our bodies won't crave quick energy because they will have healthy sources of long-lasting energy. In her book, *How to Eat to Change How You Drink,* Dr. Brooke Scheller wrote, "Protein should be incorporated at each meal and snack throughout the day and come from a variety of sources, like lean meats, seafood, eggs, dairy, nuts, seeds, beans, and legumes."[2] She explains how incorporating the right energy sources will allow you to balance your blood sugar and more effectively manage cravings for both alcohol and sugar.

I began noticing that if I started my day with protein, like eggs, instead of just a piece of toast, I would have sustained energy throughout the morning. I also began to keep high-protein snacks with me.

If, like I did, you're using sugar as a reward at the end of the day, give yourself heaps of grace and compassion initially, and remember to focus on one thing at a time. Eventually, when you feel ready, you can swap out the ice cream with lower sugar options. I switched from eating ice cream scoops to a fun, nonalcoholic drink. Four years later, I don't have massive sugar cravings in the evenings because I've slowly re-trained my body by including foods in my diet that don't spike my blood sugar. I'll still have chocolate when it sounds good, but it's not a reaction to a massive craving.

As you make healthier choices, your brain will kick-start your regular dopamine production routine again, and you'll experience fewer cravings. This is a process, and it's not linear for anyone. Be kind to yourself. Be proud of yourself for being on this journey.

A NOTE ON BODY IMAGE

It's tough to talk about food and sugar without bringing up body image. After I found freedom from alcohol, I next needed God's help with freedom from diet culture. If you picked up this book because you wanted to lose weight by not drinking, then I want you to know that for most of my life I 1,000 percent felt those feelings of wanting to be smaller and thinner. But here's the thing I learned: God called our bodies good when He created us. He loves us no matter what size we are. Unfortunately, just like getting caught up in the cultural norms of drinking, I got caught up in the cultural norms of constantly putting myself on a diet. And it's not just you and me; body image has come up in one way or another with every single client I've ever had.

Just like I had to examine my beliefs about alcohol, I had to examine my beliefs about food. Instead of making food choices in order to be a different size or according to what other people were telling me I should and shouldn't eat, I began to make food choices based on how I wanted to feel. I learned that just like I was talking to God about my stories about alcohol, I needed to talk to God about the stories surrounding my body. I needed to believe my body wasn't a constant project or something to be fixed. In her book *Breaking Free from Body Shame,* Jess Connolly wrote, "Our bodies were made and called good, and the work of our lives is not to spend the rest of our time making them acceptable, or able to measure up to whatever standard the culture has established for bodies right now."[3]

TiNA

TRY SOME THOUGHTFUL EXPERIMENTATION IN YOUR diet today by ensuring you are eating enough protein and healthy fats. How does filling up on these long-lasting sources of energy affect your sugar cravings? Get out your journal and answer this question: How can you show yourself some grace as you journey through the process of creating a life you love?

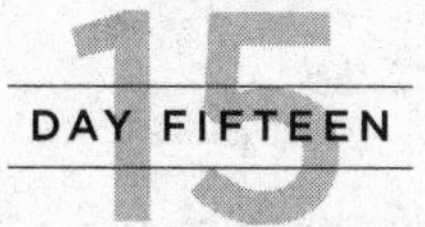

DAY FIFTEEN

Embracing Choice

May the God of hope fill you with all joy and peace as you trust in him, so that you may overflow with hope by the power of the Holy Spirit.

—ROMANS 15:13

WHEN I FIRST STARTED MY JOURNEY, I'D ONLY HEARD the overuse of alcohol referred to as a disease, which didn't help my thought process much. But there are other frameworks that help us understand why we struggle to put down that drink, which means there is more than one way to find freedom from alcohol. And *you* are the best person to decide what serves you the most.

ALCOHOL USE DISORDER (AUD)

In recent years, the medical community has been evolving its approach to alcohol addiction and now recognizes that it exists on a spectrum rather than as a one-size-fits-all disease. This understanding has led to the development of the alcohol use disorder (AUD) spectrum.[1] AUD acknowledges that the relationship with alcohol varies from person to person. It recognizes a range of behaviors, from mild to severe, which allows for a more individualized and holistic approach. This perspective highlights that there's no one way to change your relationship with alcohol, and individuals can find support and solutions that work best for them. Embracing this spectrum approach means you have choices. For me, saying I had a disordered relationship with drinking felt better than saying I had a drinking problem. But again, the choice is up to you.

THE DISEASE MODEL

The disease model suggests that alcohol addiction is a chronic disease that affects the brain, and some people are more genetically predisposed to becoming addicted to substances like alcohol.[2] If you ever hear someone say that addiction runs in their family and that's why they struggle with alcohol addiction, they're likely coming from a disease model perspective.

I've spoken to many women who say, "I'm addicted to alcohol because my relative was an alcoholic. I'm this way because of my genetics. It's just the way it is. I am stuck like this." This can be an extremely limiting belief that can cause people to live as if they are destined for misery. If this is you, stop for a second and ask yourself, "Who would I be without the thought that I am diseased?" Would it feel better to know that you have a choice and control over your decision to drink? Good news, friend: You do!

THE LEARNING MODEL

The learning model proposes that addiction is learned through experiences and associations. For example, suppose you always drink alcohol to cope with stress or anxiety. In that case, your brain learned with time to associate alcohol with relief, making it more likely for you to open a bottle of wine anytime you've had a stressful day. The learning model is one of the perspectives that has served me personally very well. As soon as I realized that my beliefs about alcohol didn't help me live the way I wanted to, I began to lose the desire to drink.

THE SELF-MEDICATION MODEL

This self-medication model suggests that people use alcohol to cope with underlying mental health issues like depression or anxiety. According to the Mayo Clinic, twice as many women as men suffer from depression.[3] As well, "From the time a girl reaches puberty until about the age of 50, she is twice as likely to have an anxiety disorder than a man. Anxiety disorders also occur earlier in women than in men."[4] This makes women more vulnerable to using alcohol as a form of self-medication.

I relate to this model a lot. When my mother died, I fell into an intense depression, and I only knew about two coping mechanisms: wine and tequila. But what I didn't realize is I was using a depressant to combat my depression, and it only made things worse. In addition to slowing down the functions of my nervous system, it dramatically affected my dopamine and serotonin neurotransmitters, exacerbating my emotions and trapping me in a cycle of alcohol use disorder.

While we may get a temporary hit of that happiness buzz produced by dopamine if we regularly drink, our overall natural levels of dopamine decrease. Since our bodies become accustomed to large artificial amounts of dopamine from alcohol, they don't need to make any on their own. This makes us feel more depressed.[5]

The self-medication and learning models go hand in hand because as soon as we dismantle the learned belief that alcohol helps depression or anxiety, we can learn that it's not an effective coping mechanism.

OPTIONS ARE EMPOWERING

Let's talk a bit more about how much choice you have when it comes to your relationship with alcohol.

I felt incredibly stuck when I was at the height of my drinking. I thought I only had two options: keep drinking and deal with the fallout *or* use willpower to quit drinking and feel deprived. The choices were bad and worse. And each day that I delayed the choice, I lived in a mental war zone of moderation, praying that I could stick to a few glasses but losing the battle repeatedly. I thought that if I was going to be miserable and always feel like I was missing out, I might as well keep drinking.

But here's more good news: There's another door. Lucky number three. And it's what we are doing here together. We have the choice and opportunity to reprogram our subconscious and step into a life of freedom and peace. In a supported break from drinking, using reflection, science, and Scripture, you can lose the desire to drink alcohol. Just like I did.

TiNA

GOD GAVE US FREE WILL TO CHOOSE HOW WE LIVE this life on earth. Spend some time in your journal today and reflect on these questions: Which model seems most empowering and helpful to you? Do you feel empowered to know that alcohol use disorder is a wide spectrum and you can choose to change, no matter how much you're drinking?

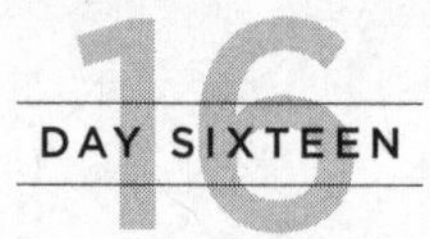

DAY SIXTEEN

The Illusion of Sleep

Come to me, all you who are weary and burdened, and I will give you rest. Take my yoke upon you and learn from me, for I am gentle and humble in heart, and you will find rest for your souls. For my yoke is easy and my burden is light.

—MATTHEW 11:28–30

SLEEP IS ESSENTIAL TO OUR HEALTH AND WELL-BEING, both mentally and physically. Matthew Walker, the world-renowned sleep scientist and author of *Why We Sleep* (a book I highly recommend), wrote, "Every major system, tissue, and organ of your body suffers when sleep becomes short. No aspect of your health can retreat at the sign of sleep loss and escape unharmed. Like water from a bust pipe in your home, the effects of sleep deprivation will seep into every nook and cranny of biology, down into your cells, even altering your most fundamental self—your DNA."[1]

Yet so many of my clients are stuck in cycles of exhaustion because of alcohol. "I used to blame it on my hormones," my Seattle-based client Julie said about her persistent tendency to wake up at three-thirty in the morning. "I also remember always picking the side of the bed closest to the door anytime we were at a hotel because I would constantly need to go to the bathroom in the middle of the night," she added. Paige, a mom of three young boys in Austin, told me that after the kids got on the school bus every morning, she went back to bed. "Every time I would go back upstairs to bed, it felt soul-destroying." I related to her so much because there were so many days where I felt lethargic, unproductive, and pretty much useless just because I had drunk too much wine the night before and didn't get a good night's sleep.

And yet, sure as the sky is blue, I believed that wine facilitated rest and particularly aided my sleep at night. It wasn't until I began experiencing genuine, undisturbed sleep, free from the crutch of alcohol, that I understood I'd had it wrong. All those hours I used to spend in bed still fell short of the authentic, restorative rest essential for my mind and body to function at their best the following day.

THE SCIENCE OF ALCOHOL AND SLEEP

In his book *Alcohol Explained,* William Porter shares that when you drink, your body only gets one or two hours of REM (rapid eye movement) sleep but that your body *needs* six or seven. Think about that for a second. You may be in bed for eight to ten hours, but your body only clocks one to two hours of quality sleep. So, you're automatically starting your day with a deficit.[2]

In *Why We Sleep,* Walker explains that alcohol is in a class of drugs called sedatives. "Alcohol sedates you out of wakefulness, but it does not induce natural sleep. The electrical brainwave state you enter via alcohol is not that of natural sleep; rather, it is akin to a light form of anesthesia," he says.[3] That's why we might feel like we've slept decently after a night of drinking; we weren't technically awake, but in reality, we were merely subjecting our brains to temporary sedation. It's like being put under anesthesia for surgery; your brain doesn't truly rest when you're put under because it's not getting the restorative REM sleep.

To compensate for the sedative effects, your brain produces stimulant chemicals, like adrenaline and cortisol, that wake you up and flood you with stress.[4] This is why you wake up at three in the morning hungover, beating yourself up for drinking too much again, and unable to get back to sleep.

And then, after that horrible night's sleep, what do we do? We guzzle coffee throughout the day. Consequently, we unknowingly engage in a tug-of-war between alcohol (a depressant and stimulant) and caffeine (even more stimulant) as they wrestle for homeostasis in our delicately designed bodies. This vicious cycle perpetuates the pattern: We consume wine to help us sleep and rely on coffee to wake us up, subjecting our bodies to an ongoing struggle for balance and ultimately leading to exhaustion.

Immediately after I stopped drinking, I slept like a dead person. I realized my body was exhausted after decades of insufficient REM sleep. After that initial phase, my sleep went a little haywire. I always tell my clients that getting into a good sleep cycle takes time. After all, if we have been drinking for decades, in many cases, our bodies may have forgotten how to make melatonin, the hormone that helps our circadian rhythm, because wine was interfering with that job.[5] So give yourself grace while your sleep resets.

Clients always, without fail, ask me, "How long does it

take for me to start sleeping properly again?" And unfortunately, all I can tell you is that God made us all different. It took a couple of months for my sleep to fully reset. For some clients it's a few weeks; for other clients it's several months. It will happen for you. Don't lose hope. Your sleep will return. You will find proper, restorative rest. And it's a game changer.

Today's verse reminds us that Jesus is the source of rest. He created the nights so we could sleep and the Sabbath for rest. He wants us to have energy and strength, to feel healthy and restored. Maybe you've already begun noticing a difference in how your body is resting; the great news is, it will continue improving from here.

TiNA

LOOK BACK ON THE LAST SIXTEEN DAYS. NOTE HOW your sleep has changed—how do you feel in the mornings, and how are your energy levels throughout the day compared to when you were drinking? Are there any other adjustments you'd like to make to your evening and morning routines to further increase the quality of your sleep, such as going to bed earlier or eliminating screen time before bed? If you haven't noticed a significant change in your sleep, I assure you it's coming. Keep going!

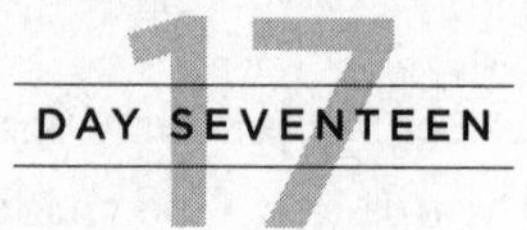

DAY SEVENTEEN

It's Not About You, It's About Them

Friends love through all kinds of weather,
and families stick together in all kinds of trouble.

—PROVERBS 17:17, MSG

After a few weeks of not drinking, I stood in the shower with hot water pouring down my back and thought about how my friends would react to the news that I wanted to take a break from alcohol. In my mind, I went through my friend groups, person by person, sorting them into two camps—the ones who would stay and the ones who would bail. I didn't know who to talk to first, and I was petrified of the reactions I might get. I didn't have one girlfriend who didn't drink.

I learned that friends and family typically have one of three kinds of reactions to sobriety.

THE MODERATION UNICORNS

First, there's the group of gals who don't care if you're not drinking because they're not hooked on alcohol. I like to call these friends the "moderation unicorns." These friends don't need alcohol to be their comforter, cheerleader, or friend. These friends could sip on one margarita at dinner and not even notice if they don't finish it. These women, in my experience, are few and far between because of the fact that it is very difficult to moderate alcohol. They are utterly unconcerned with your drinking because they are entirely unconcerned with their own drinking.

My friend Lauren is a moderation unicorn. I remember being almost fixated on how she could have one glass of wine at a girls' dinner. When I ditched alcohol, I had so many questions for her. After a few conversations, it became obvious that Lauren did not think about alcohol like I did. It didn't consume her thoughts, and it wasn't calling any shots in her life. Lauren wasn't giving any jobs to alcohol. She simply ordered the glass because of societal conditioning (i.e., everyone else was having one). When I told her I was no longer drinking, she was surprised, but the conversation quickly moved on to another topic. You'll probably experience similar scenarios with your moderation unicorn friends.

THE LOVE-YOU-NO-MATTER-WHATS

The second camp is the Love-You-No-Matter-Whats. These friends will be surprised that you're turning down a glass of wine because it's a new behavior for you. They may ask questions and prod at your reasoning, but in the end, they will support your decision because they love you.

My friend Kendra and I used to love to drink together. Whenever we hung out, alcohol was involved. I wasn't sure which camp she was going to fall into. I knew Kendra wouldn't fall into the moderation unicorn group since she drank as I did. Yet, when I told her I was taking a break, she was the first to suggest other things we could do instead of drinking. We started meeting for walks in the park, and she introduced me to the game of padel and asked me to join her padel group. Kendra became curious and asked me questions about my journey. Our relationship did the opposite of what I feared would happen; our bond grew stronger instead of breaking.

These first two groups are the women who will continue to stand by you and find reasons to hang out that don't always involve barhopping or wine tasting. It's also possible, like it was for me, that more women will fall into these two groups than you had originally anticipated.

MIRROR GAZERS

Then there is the third group of "mirror gazers," who you're likely most nervous about. These friends' reaction to your lack of drinking alcohol is more about them than about you. Here's what I mean: When you announce you're not drinking, that friend wonders if they need to take a break from alcohol too. In one mental leap, they fear that they might be classified as an alcoholic. We know the stigma of these labels—even if the word is never spoken aloud, the idea of it carries weight. The mirror gazer may consider sobriety to be a fate worse than death. Even though this may not be your intention, you are holding up a mirror and making her question her own drinking. And not everyone likes that. So this friend might have an opinion about you ordering a mocktail and vocalize it to you.

At one point, I was a big-time mirror gazer. Before I

stopped drinking, one of my best friends decided to take a monthlong break from drinking. "I'm having a sober September," she said. We'd been drinking together all summer, and she wanted to give her body a break. I remember giving her the hardest time about it. I told her the decision was silly. "Why take a month off? We have your birthday this month!" I was *not* kind. I pressured and needled her. I was rude because I worried what her decision meant for me: I was scared that if she took a break from drinking, it might mean that I also had to. I was afraid to lose one of my main drinking partners. Do you see how I made it all about me? It had nothing to do with her and her decision not to drink. I've since gone back and apologized to my friend.

When you're worried about someone giving you a hard time about not drinking, remember that friend is likely more concerned about their own drinking than yours.

When I stopped drinking, one or two ladies fell into this third camp of women. They didn't support my decision. At first I was a little hurt, but now I see it as a huge blessing. I know which friendships are authentic and which are based on drinking. This realization took time, but as we proceed on our journey and continue to learn, we get stronger and more mentally clear about friendships. Trust me on this one.

Worrying about what other people thought kept me stuck in the drinking cycle longer than I needed to be. If I could do it again, I would have started my break from alcohol sooner and not worried over what other people thought about my decision.

If you experience pushback from friends or family, remember to stay firm. Taking a break from alcohol is one of the best decisions you can make for your health and, yes, your relationships. This is a decision to be celebrated, not criticized. With that said, here are some helpful tips for navigating tricky conversations.

FLIP THE SCRIPT

One way to help ease the fears about what other people will think is to put the shoe on the other foot for a minute. I just did this in a session with a client. Carrie was worried about meeting up with a friend she hadn't seen in a while. "She is one of my friends I have drunk with since university," she explained. Carrie was considering ordering a drink to make her friend feel comfortable. Carrie assumed if she didn't, her friend would feel a certain way about her and her decision.

I said, "Put yourself in your friend's shoes for a second. What if she was taking a break from alcohol, but she had a drink with you anyways, just so you wouldn't feel bad. Would you want your friend to drink a substance with known health risks, including direct links to cancer, to make you feel comfortable?"

"I would feel awful," Carrie said. "I wouldn't ever want anyone to have a drink to make me feel better."

I smiled and said what Carrie already knew was coming: "Then why would you have a drink for her to make her feel a certain way?"

THE ART OF SAYING NO

Saying no to alcohol can be challenging, especially when you're used to indulging in social drinking. But the more you flex your boundary muscle, the easier it becomes to say no. The key is to have an answer prepared.

Avoid excuses that aren't true for you, like saying, "I'm on antibiotics" or "I'm training for a marathon." Honesty is always the best policy; most people will respect you for telling the truth. For example, if you're at a party and someone offers you a drink, reply with a positive response rather than a negative one. Saying yes instead of no can help empower you. So, instead of declining when someone offers you a drink, say something like, "Sure, I'll take a sparkling water" (or whatever your favorite alcohol-free drink might be).

If you do get asked a follow-up question, it's best to be prepared with an authentic answer. Here are a few responses that can help you avoid any further questioning. They might even lead to healthy conversations and deeper connections with your friends.

"I'm taking a break."
"I feel better when I don't drink."
"I want to get a good night's sleep tonight."
"I'm focusing on my health right now."
"I'm done with hangovers."
"I'm much more relaxed when I don't drink."
"Drinking increases my anxiety."

These responses are simple, honest, and straightforward. What would you add to this list?

TiNA

BEGIN PRACTICING THE ART OF SAYING NO TO alcohol. Circle a response or two from the list on the previous page that you will use at your next social event, or write down a few of your own. It takes time, but you'll begin to feel more empowered and in control of your choices each time you stand firm in your commitment.

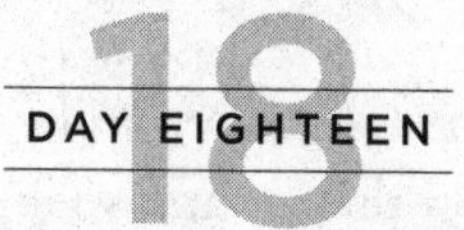

DAY EIGHTEEN

Boundaries Are Your Best Friend

> *Do not be deceived: God is not mocked, for whatever one sows, that will he also reap. For the one who sows to his own flesh will from the flesh reap corruption, but the one who sows to the Spirit will from the Spirit reap eternal life.*
>
> —GALATIANS 6:7–8, ESV

BECAUSE I STARTED MY ALCOHOL FAST DURING THE PANDEMIC, it was a few months before I had a social gathering to attend—a small Fourth of July barbecue. I was petrified of what it would feel like to turn down the rosé among friends I had been drinking with for many years. I knew in those early days that I would need to set a clear boundary of how long I would be at this party to avoid making the whole situation more difficult on myself. The party started at noon, and I told Chris I would like to head home by six. When it was time to leave, we started saying our goodbyes. Friend after friend tried to get us to stay longer. I had expected those responses, but it was still hard.

Our car was blocked by another friend's car, who half-jokingly refused to move it as a way to get us to stay. Our two kids also begged and pleaded to stay, making the whole exit even more difficult. Finally, after multiple attempts, we were able to leave. I got in the car and sobbed all the way home. This was my very first attempt at flexing my boundary muscle, and I felt like I had failed. I thought I would have to live like a hermit forever.

Three months later, we had a fortieth birthday party for Ava, one of my closest friends. I had been to several social events at that point and still always set a time to leave. The party included cocktails at a swanky new London hotel rooftop bar followed by dinner at a members' club in Mayfair. After dinner, the plan was to go back to a hotel room for more drinks and dancing. I knew the dinner would end around eleven, which would be my cue to leave. Even though drinking Christy used to love—and I do mean *love*—a late-night dance party, I knew heading home after dinner was what I wanted to do.

After dinner, as we stepped outside the restaurant, I looked into Ava's eyes and said, "I am going home." She looked at me with a small frown and then gave me a massive hug. She told me she understood. I got in the car and cried again, but this time they were tears of relief. *I can do this,* I thought. I had been there for the best part, where I got to celebrate and connect with the birthday girl, and that's what mattered. Whether you're a people pleaser like me or someone who fears missing out on the fun, sticking to your boundaries can help you live intentionally and fall in love with your life again.

One of the most important things we can learn while on an alcohol fast is to set these boundaries. For example, when I first told Chris I needed to take a break from alcohol, I asked him if he could please not drink at home until I had a better handle on things. That was one of the most important boundaries I've ever asked for, and I am so grateful he honored it for those first few months as I navigated my way through.

A huge gift in going alcohol-free has been the realization that I don't have to live my life for other people. I want to live my life for Jesus and my family. I get to decide how to spend my time, money, and energy. I no longer want to spend these precious God-given resources on making other people happy.

COMMUNICATION AND CONSISTENT ACTION

Setting boundaries requires two things: communication and consistent action. If we don't communicate what we need (e.g., "I am leaving the party now" or "I need the wine out of the house"), then we might wind up feeling bitter or responding in a passive-aggressive way. When we can clearly articulate our boundaries, we are less likely to be misunderstood.[1]

Once our boundary has been communicated, we must maintain it consistently. I struggled in the beginning with setting boundaries with friends because no one had ever heard them before or seen me stand by them. I used to be famous for saying, "I'm going out for just one drink," and then sneaking back into the house long after the kids had gone to bed. I never stuck to my plans. That's why when I began to communicate my boundaries and consistently abide by them, people were surprised.

After about a year of living alcohol-free, I attended a girls'-night-out dinner. When the server asked me what I wanted to drink, I picked up the menu, flipped to the mocktail section, and casually picked one. That scenario in the first few months of not drinking would have made me nervous, but I'd had practice. It had become second nature. It was easy. I knew I felt so much better without alcohol, so at that point, I wouldn't have cared if anyone said anything about me not drinking. But on this occasion, no one was surprised. My not-drinking boundary was clear.

Remember, practice makes perfect. The first few times you set boundaries will probably feel scary and unfamiliar, but pay attention to how setting and sticking to your intentions feels instead of getting caught up in what other people may or may not think. I promise this gets easier, my beautiful friend.

NO APOLOGIES OR EXPLANATIONS REQUIRED

In those early days of not drinking, I did a lot of apologizing for leaving events or gatherings early. But I knew if I didn't leave at my decided time, I would be exhausted the next day, skip my early morning prayer time, be grumpy with the kids, and find long days of work difficult. To me, not getting adequate rest felt similar to a hangover. After some time, I realized I didn't have to apologize for doing what was best for me.

We also don't need to explain why we are setting a boundary, just like we don't have to give a long answer for turning down a drink. "No" is a perfectly fine answer. We don't have to justify or over-explain wanting to do what's best for our health.

In today's verses, Paul talks about how we reap what we sow. We have to set boundaries and work at something to get the desired outcome. The goals of feeling better, having more patience, getting your joy back, and sleeping better are more than worth the effort.

In her book *Chase the Fun,* Annie F. Downs wrote, "If you are tired, no is a complete sentence. It will allow you the rest you need. If you are feeling burned out, no is a complete sentence. It will allow you a chance to refuel. If you are feeling too busy, no is a complete sentence. It will open up space for what matters most. If you just don't want to, no is a complete sentence. It will help you be a good friend to yourself."[2]

TiNA

WHAT BOUNDARIES HAVE YOU PUT INTO PRACTICE already that have helped you stay on track with your alcohol fast? Consider what other boundaries you might put into effect to help you even more. Write them down in a journal or record them in a note on your phone so you have them handy.

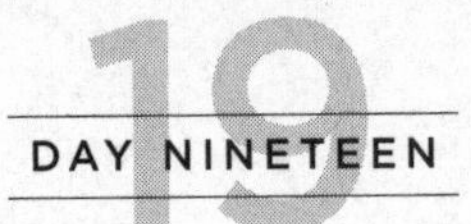

DAY NINETEEN

Joyful Movement

She dresses herself with strength
and makes her arms strong.

—PROVERBS 31:17, ESV

ONE OF THE MOST CRITICAL COMPONENTS IN HELPING me break free from alcohol was moving my body in a way that felt really good. You may be thinking, *Christy, you said on day one that I didn't have to dive into a new workout routine; why are you talking to me about exercise?* Today, I want to talk about exercise *not* as a way to change your body or how it looks but as an essential tool to boost your mood, help with cravings, relieve boredom, help you sleep better, and improve your emotional and mental health.

BOOST YOUR MOOD

Here's my chance to quote Elle Woods from *Legally Blonde* (although I'm wary of the word *exercise,* and I'll soon explain why): When defending a fitness instructor who is being accused of murder, law student Elle says, "Exercise gives you endorphins. Endorphins make you happy. Happy people just don't shoot their husbands. They just don't."[1] And you can't argue with that. Endorphins naturally boost our mood, reduce the feeling of pain, and increase feelings of pleasure. Combining endorphins and dopamine by moving our bodies is a surefire way to get us feeling better, whereas drinking negatively affects the production of both neurotransmitters because while we may get an immediate high, the fallout after the initial increase lowers our mood.[2]

I used to believe drinking helped my feelings of anxiety, but in reality, drinking increases our cortisol levels, making us feel more anxious and depressed.[3] Moving our bodies lowers our cortisol levels, which naturally gives us the relief we seek.[4]

However, if, like me, you have been associating exercise with punishing your body for the food you ate or how much you drank or because it's long been an ongoing project to get skinnier and stay that way, then you may have to reframe the whole concept of exercise as something that makes you feel good.

I removed the word *exercise* from my vocabulary altogether. It had too many negative connotations for me. Instead, I talk about how I joyfully move my body.

CURB YOUR CRAVINGS

Moving our bodies is also a great way to get cravings under control. When you get an urge, one of the first things to consider is what you are looking for in that glass of wine. If it's relief from stress, moving your body is one of the most effective ways to do so. If you're craving rest, gentle movement will help you sleep better. If you're bored, movement will give you something fun to do. If you're searching for connection, walking or hiking with a friend or family member is a beautiful way to feel better and make memories together. We can literally move our body through a temporary craving and feel better on the other side.

KEEP IT SIMPLE

Never underestimate the power of a good walk outside. When I began my alcohol fast, I spent a lot of time walking. We were in the middle of a pandemic, and here in the UK we were allowed to visit our local park once a day. So I walked and walked and walked. I listened to podcasts, books, sermons, and music while I moved my body. Even though I was stuck inside most of the time, homeschooling two kiddos and living with a lawyer husband who was clocking even more hours at home than he had in the office, I could regulate my mood by walking.

I used to think I had to carve out at least an hour every day for a strenuous workout, but those lockdown walks taught me differently. When I changed the focus from calorie burning to better mental health, I learned that even a ten-minute dance party around the kitchen island boosted my mood immensely. As the saying goes, every little bit helps.

You decide how best to move your body and for how long. The choice is yours.

Add Prayer to the Movement

I've found a Pilates studio nearby that I love. The feeling of doing Pilates helps me connect to my body, and the slow-paced movement allows me to also pray simultaneously or spend some quiet time in thought.

Is there a gentle, joyful movement that you really enjoy? Try to incorporate prayer in that time this week and see how it can positively impact your mood and perspective for your day. Pilates and prayer or walking and prayer are great combinations for me. What might work well for you?

Movement and Community

Another way to make movement fun is to add friends. I mentioned this earlier, but during my first year of sobriety, I started playing padel. I also got to know some of the ladies in my Pilates class and would meet them for walks or coffee. Participating in a group sport or class is a fantastic way to integrate both movement and a sense of community.

If you find solitary movement tedious, why not try something a bit more social? Other racket sports like tennis, pickleball, or paddle tennis are fun. What about barre or a dance class? Again, experiment and find what you enjoy. Use this opportunity to figure out what lights you up and makes you feel that endorphin spike without worrying about how many calories you're burning.

Get Motivated

Don't get me wrong; there are days when I don't want to move. But since I shifted the way I think about exercise—moving my body for my mental and emotional health instead of to punish myself or to fix my body—it is less of a battle. But when we have a low-motivation day, I encourage you to use the play-the-tape-forward tactic in a slightly different way.

Fast-forward the tape to the end of the workout or class or walk and think about how you will feel. Are you glad you went, or do you wish you had stayed on the couch? Has the walk or workout helped your mood? Has it given you more energy today, and might it allow you to sleep better tonight? Remembering how you will feel *after* moving your body helps you recognize the benefits. And if you have days where movement would truly drain you more than lift you up, then skip it. Remember, rest is just as important as moving your body. Above all, be kind to yourself. Ask yourself what your body really needs. Grace and compassion are key here.

TiNA

YEP, YOU GUESSED IT. YOUR TINY NEW ACTION TODAY is to move your body, even if it's just for ten minutes. Move your body, even if it's a dance party around the kitchen island with your kiddos or a few simple stretches on the floor. Pay attention to how you feel before and afterward.

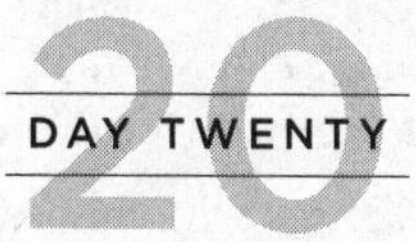

DAY TWENTY

The Power of Gratitude

Oh give thanks to the LORD, *for he is good;*
for his steadfast love endures forever!

—1 CHRONICLES 16:34, ESV

DURING THE CHALLENGING DAYS OF THE COVID-19 LOCKdown, our unique situation, living as expats in the UK with concerns about potential border closures, added to our stress. At first, we didn't feel comfortable flying back to the US for fear of getting Covid en route and sharing it with family members. When the restrictions were relaxed for the first time, we rented a small cottage in the middle of nowhere in Yorkshire to get out of the big city and have a little open space. After a five-hour drive, we arrived. Nothing much changed about our day-to-day routine: Chris was still working insane hours for his law firm, and the kids were being homeschooled via their school iPads. I was working and focusing on staying alcohol-free.

I'll never forget that first walk I took alone in Yorkshire. The sun was shining while Copper and I strolled through fields and forests. I prayed as I wandered, thanking God for the opportunity to get out of the city, for the sunshine, for the local farmers market, for our family's health, and for the new path I was on. We were in the middle of a global pandemic, yet my heart was overcome with gratitude.

I realized that when I used wine to numb the stress of life, I was also numbing my ability to see blessings. Drinking had completely taken my focus off all the incredible things God had provided for my family and me. Gratitude slowly but surely became an essential tool in my sobriety toolkit.

THE SCIENCE OF GRATITUDE

Many studies have concluded that gratitude has real, tangible benefits for our bodies and mental health. It makes us happier and more resilient. Practicing gratitude improves blood pressure.[1] It increases our dopamine and serotonin, neurotransmitters responsible for helping us feel happier. It also lowers cortisol, the stress hormone. The combined effect of gratitude in our neurochemistry reduces both anxiety and depression.[2]

GRATITUDE INCREASES PATIENCE

Focusing on my blessings and not suffering from a constant low-grade hangover meant I was more patient. Instead of getting frustrated by London traffic, I began feeling so grateful that I could listen to podcasts and worship music in the car and have that space and time to pray and learn from God. Instead of getting frustrated with my children because they hadn't cleaned up their rooms, I shifted to an attitude of gratefulness because of the realization that time was flying and I wouldn't have messy kids living at home with me forever.

A regular practice of gratitude changed my mindset; gradually, there were fewer and fewer reasons to want to check out with a glass of wine. I went from being completely stressed about my life to having zero desire to escape because I recognized how many good things were all around me.

GRATITUDE FOR LESSONS LEARNED

I used to carry around so much shame about things I did while drinking. There were evenings when I neglected my children because I'd rather drink wine than read them a bedtime story. There were unhelpful text messages to family members I never would have sent if I hadn't been drinking. But all those instances when I disappointed myself and let myself down taught me that wine wasn't the answer. All the events on my sobriety journey led me to write this book; so instead of feeling ashamed, I now thank God for the journey. Romans 5:3–5 says we should "rejoice in our sufferings, knowing that suffering produces endurance, and endurance produces character, and character produces hope, and hope does not put us to shame" (ESV). He allows us to go through trials and difficult situations so that we learn to rely on and find ultimate hope in Him. This journey you're on right now may feel heavy and hard, but it can lead to freedom. That's something to be so grateful for.

GRATITUDE GIVES PERSPECTIVE

The Bible tells us to be thankful not only because God created us and blessed us with so many things but most importantly because He gave His Son's life for us so that we could have peace, hope, and eternal life. First Thessalonians 5:16–18 reads, "Be cheerful no matter what; pray all the time; thank God no matter what happens. This is the way God wants you who belong to Christ Jesus to live" (MSG). In this passage, Paul encourages Christians to give thanks even when faced with hardship and adversity, as it helps us to maintain a positive outlook and to focus on the things that truly matter. I know this isn't always easy, my beautiful friend, but it's something we can strive for, and the Holy Spirit will help us along the way.

When I was drinking, the gospel was not at the forefront of my mind because I wasn't spending time each day in prayer and thankfulness to God for what He had done in my life. Living alcohol-free has reminded me what this life is all about. I shouldn't look for a way to go numb if I've had a bad day, because God is the ultimate Comforter (2 Corinthians 1:3–4). As humans, we are quick to reach for creature comforts that bring fleeting relief, often with consequences. But when we seek comfort in the almighty Comforter, He provides true peace. When I start my day thanking and praising God, it brings a great perspective to my life.

Concentrating on what you are grateful for takes the focus off your fears and anxiety. Again, it's about taking your thoughts captive and figuring out what is true. When you're not focused on fear and anxiety, there are fewer negative thoughts in your mind to lead you to a place where you want to go numb. When you begin living your life with gratitude and intention, you will rediscover a life you genuinely love that requires no escape with alcohol.

BUILDING A GRATITUDE PRACTICE

Cultivating a gratitude practice is simple. Here are a few ideas to get you started.

- Start your prayers by thanking God for any good things in your life, big or small. Psalm 100:4 says, "Enter his gates with thanksgiving." I love to start my conversations with God by thanking Him for everything He has blessed me with, and I try to remember to thank Him for the prayers He has answered. When I journal my prayer requests, it's easy to go back and see all the prayers God answered.
- Keep a daily gratitude journal. Write down three things that you are grateful for each day. These add up with a little time, and it's so encouraging to go back occasionally to review how many gifts God has given.
- At the dinner table, ask those you're sharing a meal with—your family or friends—what they're thankful for that day. I'm working on making this part of our routine at home, going around the table and sharing what we're grateful for a couple times a week.
- You can also write letters of gratitude to friends and family to tell them how grateful you are that God placed them in your life. This is an incredible way to deepen your connections with those you love.

Cultivating gratitude may take time, but it's so worth it. When we build in these practices, we'll see our outlook and perspective change.

TiNA

PICK ONE SUGGESTION ABOVE TO INCORPORATE INTO your daily or weekly routine. Whether starting your prayers with thanksgiving or starting a daily gratitude journal, the practice of gratitude will enable you to fall in love with your life again and give you fewer reasons to escape or numb with alcohol.

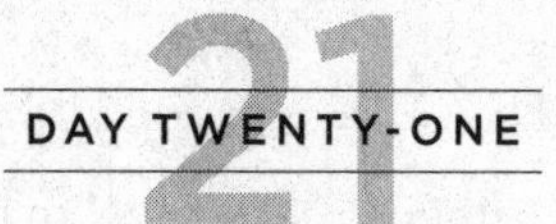

DAY TWENTY-ONE

Redefining Self-Care

Be still, and know that I am God.

—PSALM 46:10

ONE OF THE MOST PERVASIVE MESSAGES WE FACE IN our society—especially as women—is that drinking is a form of self-care. The amount of information we have in our subconscious filing cabinets to support this story is overwhelming. But the truth is that regular drinking leads to headaches, hangovers, and health risks. We entirely disregard our future selves when we drink. Drinking alcohol isn't self-care; it's self-sabotage.

We need a better way to take care of ourselves—true self-care. I love how Amanda E. White explained it:

> Contrary to popular belief, most real self-care isn't Instagram-able. It's not glamorous. It's not "treating yourself" or something you can buy. Self-care is going to the dentist when you've been avoiding it, saying no to a trip you can't afford, turning off your phone, or drinking a glass of water. People do not have to earn their right to practice self-care, just as they don't have to earn their

> right to go to sleep each night. Rest and self-care are necessary, and it's impossible for [us] to be mentally well or to regulate emotions if [we] aren't taking care of ourselves.[1]

Instagram will tell us that self-care is shopping or getting your nails done, but it can also mean making a healthy, nourishing meal at home, or working on your family budget. It might mean moving your body, even if it's just fifteen minutes of stretching. It also might mean skipping your workout and napping if your body needs it. It's going to look different for each of us. It's care and concern for your future self, not just the immediate gratification of something quick to numb you or quickly change your emotional state.

The Bible is clear about taking care of ourselves. Paul wrote in 1 Corinthians 6:19–20: "Do you not know that your bodies are temples of the Holy Spirit, who is in you, whom you have received from God? You are not your own; you were bought at a price. Therefore honor God with your bodies." This scripture drives home the point that we must care for brains and bodies in a way that truly reflects and aligns with our relationship with God.

BE STILL

As today's verse prompts us to remember, sometimes self-care is about being still and knowing God is at the wheel. Sometimes the most meaningful rest comes when I turn off the music, shut off the podcasts, and sit in quiet reflection, knowing that God's plan is unfolding as it should. I don't have to physically or mentally strive any harder for His plan to become reality.

Sitting with God at five in the morning with a cup of hot coffee is the best thing I can do to help my stress, anxiety, and overwhelm. I like to think of this time as "soul care," an essential part of my self-care routine. For me, soul care incorporates gratitude, prayer, and meditating on truth. If you're skipping soul care, then I encourage you to carve out time in your busy schedule for this essential piece of self-care.

Try this prayerful breathing exercise. Read just the first line of Psalm 46:10, incorporating slow, deep breaths as you slowly break down the verse, word by word.

Say "Be still, and know that I am God . . ." Take a deep breath in for four seconds, then exhale for six seconds.

Say "Be still, and know that I am . . ." Take a deep breath in for four seconds, then exhale for six seconds.

Say "Be still, and know . . ." Take a deep breath in for four seconds, then exhale for six seconds.

Say "Be still . . ." Take a deep breath in for four seconds, then exhale for six seconds.

Say "Be . . ." Take a deep breath in for four seconds, then exhale for six seconds.

Once you get the hang of it, this is a prayerful breathing exercise you can use whenever you feel overwhelmed.

TRUE REST

One of the most essential parts of soul care is rest. God created the Sabbath to give us this reminder, yet we often forget how important rest is.[2] We need rest, and if we don't get it in ways that serve us, we turn to less healthy, less satisfying methods like alcohol for a false form of rest. We've already talked about how alcohol destroys our sleep, but real rest and soul care goes much deeper than sleep.

Weekends are no longer rest time for me. If you're a mom, you know what I mean. Weekends mean sports practices, dance classes, birthday parties, and playdates. But I've figured out how to carve out some time for rest after my children head to school on Monday morning. I don't meet with clients then; I usually try to make sure I go for a long walk or take a Pilates class. I had to get intentional and plan out this time for rest to stave off feeling overwhelmed on Saturdays when I'm driving all over town between Ella's drama practices and Carter's basketball games.

My client Jessica in St. Louis is a single mom of four who works as a full-time nurse. Her only form of self-care after a long day of work and caring for the kids was drinking. Together, we got intentional about her self-care schedule. Every week, we would look ahead and ensure she had time for herself. This meant doing her weekly budgeting on Monday, taking a walk on her lunch break, and turning her phone off at eight o'clock in the evening so she could go to bed by nine. This might not look like the self-care we see promoted on social media, but these small changes gave Jessica more quality rest and peace of mind than a bottle of wine.

What works for Jessica and me may not work for you. It's

all about finding the tools that work best for *your* life. I recommend curiosity and experimentation here. Don't be discouraged if it takes a few tries to identify the small tweaks that deeply impact your self-care.

TiNA

THIS FAST IS ABOUT DESIGNING A LIFE YOU LOVE, A life you don't want to escape from. Take out your calendar and schedule some time for self-care this week. Remember, it doesn't have to be long or idyllic. Block off time at least once or twice a week to take a break. Even if it's just a nap or walking the dog and listening to worship music, ensure you create time for some life-giving activity. Try to incorporate soul care into your daily routine, even if it's just a few minutes.

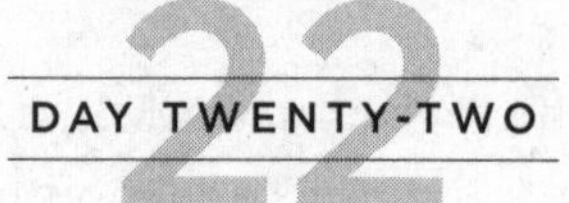

DAY TWENTY-TWO

New Ways to Cope

The Lord is near to the brokenhearted
and saves the crushed in spirit.

—PSALM 34:18, ESV

I'VE ALREADY SHARED HOW MY MOM'S DEATH GREATLY impacted my drinking, but I haven't explained yet how alcohol slowly but surely took over as my main coping mechanism.

On March 9, 2018, I was getting ready to go out to dinner when I got a call from my younger brother, David. "Mom died."

I think I started screaming, "No!" I fell on the bathroom floor. I texted two of my closest girlfriends, who were at my house in minutes. One of them called Virgin Atlantic to book a flight for me, and the other packed my suitcase.

I had done that flight from London to Los Angeles dozens of times, but this one was awful. I asked for a glass of wine when we were in the air. I drank for eleven straight hours. I don't remember watching any television or movies on the flight. I am not sure how I wound up at my dad's house. It's all a blur.

I walked into my parents' kitchen, and there on the refrigerator door was a note written by my mom: "Christy and the kids arrive March 17th at 3:10. LAX." We had planned to visit for Easter. I had missed her by just eight days.

Over the following weeks I planned my mother's funeral, picked the urn to store her cremated ashes, and wrote her obituary. I drank through all of it. I also picked up vaping. Chris and the kids arrived for the funeral. After the service, I spent weeks in LA drinking rosé during the day and red wine at night. Ella and Carter mostly hung out with a babysitter. No one questioned anything I was doing; my mother had just died.

Once the kids' spring break was over, we returned to London. I met up with two girlfriends at my local pub. It was lunchtime, and we ordered a bottle of wine. I told them how horrible the entire trip was, how I wanted to speak at the funeral but couldn't. After I tearfully recalled the memories of the past month, I looked at the almost empty bottle of wine on the table and said, "I know it's probably early to be drinking this much."

"You have a year," said one of my friends, who had also lost her mother. "Do what you need to do."

So I did. I hit the self-destruct button. When I was home alone, I would drink until I cried. When I was out, I would drink until the early morning hours. I preferred being out to being home because it meant my children didn't see me acting like a mess. My relationship with Chris was in tatters; I felt like he didn't understand me. I felt alone. I barely spoke to God, not because I was angry at Him for taking my mom, but because I thought He surely was ashamed of my behavior. What kind of Christian was I? No one on the outside would ever have known I had a relationship with Him.

I woke up with a nasty hangover one morning, remembering I had a lunch date with a girlfriend who wouldn't think twice if I suggested a bottle of rosé. *If I can just get to lunch, I can open that bottle. Then I'll feel better,* I thought. I remember a tiny alarm bell going off in my brain. *That can't be good,* it said. But nothing changed.

It sounds like I was drinking a lot, and I was, but here's the thing: It didn't look much different from how everyone around me seemed to be drinking. Every mom I knew had a glass of wine or two at night. To the outside world, I looked like I had it all together. I was on time for school pickup. I was on the PTA. I had a successful lifestyle blog about my "glamorous" London life. I kept up the perfect Instagram facade, carefully choosing which photos to share with the world. No one ever mentioned that I might be drinking too much. So I kept going. Until that day in March 2020, two years after my mom's death. I'd had enough.

I didn't want to spend another year feeling this way. Broken. Exhausted. Devastated. Alone. I realized that drinking wasn't going to fix my grief. Only Jesus could do that job. And so I surrendered all of it to Him. I began begging Him for forgiveness and the supernatural healing and peace that only He could provide.

The grief I was coping with had many levels. I was angry at my mom for choosing alcohol over me. I was devastated that she was taken so soon. I felt like no one could understand what I was going through. But I realized that God did. He knows all about losing someone He loves, His only Son. He could fill that hole in my heart like no one else could, and He could also help me to forgive my mom.

I have had the privilege of coaching numerous women who had turned to alcohol to cope with grief. Grief arises from a variety of circumstances—from the loss of a loved one, chronic pain, a wayward child, illness, missed opportunities, and so many more. Society often conditions us to believe that alcohol provides solace, but I truthfully tell you that it does not.

The journey to healing from grief is a process. Numbing with alcohol blocks this process. Although I still experience sadness on some days, my grief has transformed significantly. Psalm 147:3 says "He heals the brokenhearted and binds up their wounds." Reflecting back, I see God's hand in every moment of my journey. In her book *WayMaker,* Ann Voskamp wrote, "Life is waves. Grief comes in waves. Suffering comes in waves. Losses come in waves. There is no controlling life's storms; there is only learning to live with waves. The real work of being human is mastering how to process losses while being in the process of moving forward. The real work of being human is trusting the way is the waves, right through the valleys and crests. Across the waves, even now right now, the Spirit hovers."[1] What waves have you experienced recently?

God was by my side throughout my grief—whether I was crying out to Him in drunken despair, weeping through a hangover, or, finally, surrendering it all to Him. Life has presented its challenges after my mother's passing, but God has taught me that He constantly shows up with a plan. I just have to trust in Him and ride the waves. If you're experiencing grief right now, I want you to know that the Holy Spirit is with you, offering comfort and peace that surpasses anything alcohol could ever provide.

GRIEVING THE OLD YOU

Another aspect of grief that isn't talked about very much in sobriety circles is mourning the loss of your identity as a drinker. Whether you've been known as the "*hostess with the mostest*" or the "*life and soul of the party,*" it can be challenging to fully realize who you are now without alcohol and who God is shaping you to become until you navigate the "death" of the person you identified as before.

I remember feeling a heaviness the first few times I left a social event without drinking. There was this awkward unexplainable grief wrapped up in the dissonance of knowing I didn't want to stay late but still wanting to be the girl who shuts the party down. The last woman standing. The girl who always suggests, "Just one more glass."

Now I know. I was grieving a party-girl Christy, knowing I wanted to become a better version of myself without any vision of what that new version looked like. It was a suffocating feeling of not knowing who I was but knowing I could do better. It was the sadness of leaving a big piece of who I thought I was without being able to see who I would become.

If you have that nagging feeling that you were meant for more than a life of hangovers, if there's a piece of you that knows deep down that wine is holding you back, then I want to be honest with you: Parts of this journey are messy. But the encouraging part is that the messy parts don't last forever. The encouraging part is that the woman you get to grow into and become, the one who God has called you to be, is someone you'll want to meet. She's confident. She's fun. She's full of purpose. She's waiting for you.

TiNA

IF YOU'VE USED ALCOHOL AS A COPING MECHANISM for grief, loss, or disappointment, then you are not alone. Here are a few journaling ideas: List the significant losses you've experienced thus far in your life. What have been your default coping mechanisms? What have you learned about yourself and who God is from these hard times? What things are true about God that makes the grief you're feeling more bearable? Has alcohol truly helped in healing? However you might answer these questions, I encourage you to spend some time in prayer after journaling. God doesn't mind tears or honest words.

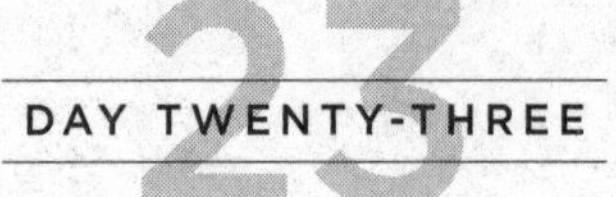

DAY TWENTY-THREE

A Change of Taste

Praise the Lord, *my soul;*
all my inmost being, praise his holy name.
Praise the Lord, *my soul,*
and forget not all his benefits . . .
who satisfies your desires with good things
so that your youth is renewed like the eagle's.

—PSALM 103:1–2, 5

In London, we have a real rat problem. I know, it's gross. There are rats all over the city, and I don't have one friend who hasn't had to deal with them at some point or another. Our house has a little attached side room that we call the scooter closet because it stores the kids' scooters and bikes. One morning, I walked into our kitchen and almost gagged from the smell. After a panicked call to the exterminator, we found that a rat had died in the scooter closet and the smell permeated the house.

The problem was we couldn't get to the rat's body because it was somewhere in the pipes under the floor. So the exterminator told us we would have to live with the smell for a week or so. It was disgusting. I cried. But then I went on Amazon and found all sorts of deodorizing bags and smell-blocking plug-ins. After a couple of days, I couldn't smell it anymore. The kids stopped complaining about it. We could start eating in the kitchen again because the smell didn't bother us.

It wasn't until we had friends walk into our house and shout, "Oh my gosh, what is that smell?" that I realized our sense of smell had adapted. The foul smell was still there; we just weren't offended by it anymore.

All our senses adjust with time and exposure. We become accustomed to alcohol by drinking it over and over. Most of us didn't like the taste of wine or any other alcohol when we first tried it, but over time—with a ton of societal pressure telling us we *should* like it—we eventually did. We started finding it palatable and slowly began enjoying the taste. But, when we give our taste buds a little time off from drinking alcohol and start realizing how it truly makes us feel, we can again lose the taste for it.

The first time that I tried alcohol, I was sixteen. I was at my best friend Holly's house, whose mom was a flight attendant and was out of town for work. We had the brilliant idea of trying tequila. We didn't even attempt to mix it, we went straight into doing shots, re-creating what we had seen on MTV's Spring Break. Lick the salt, slam the shot, and grab the lime. It tasted awful, and obviously we felt so sick. I did not see the appeal of the taste of alcohol at all, and yet this seemed like what we were supposed to be doing to fit in and be "cool."

Years later, when I met my husband, Chris, in law school, we started learning about wine. We went to Napa together, and later when we studied law in London, we took trips to France and Italy, sampling and collecting wine along the way. We dreamed of the day we would have children and how we would start wine cellars for each of them.

We became wine snobs. We loved to find restaurants with tasting menus to sample different varietals of wine. We bought fancy decanters and glassware. After we were engaged, my godmother threw us a bar shower, a wedding shower where everyone brought stuff for your bar. We got dozens of sets of fancy glassware, books about cocktail-making, embroidered cocktail napkins, and bottles upon bottles of wine.

So, how did I go from a sixteen-year-old girl thinking the taste of alcohol was disgusting to drinking wine as a main hobby? It comes down to conditioning. I firmly believed enjoying the taste of alcohol was sophisticated because of what I had seen, heard, and experienced over many years. The world had taught me that the taste of alcohol was good. But is this really true?

Heidi, one of my clients, told me how she loved the taste of beer. She was very interested in the craft brewing scene. In one of our sessions I challenged her, "What if, at the end of the day when you sit out on your back porch, you try an alcohol-free beer instead?" I listed the names of several brands. She looked at me and said, "But that's just not the same." I responded, "But if you're drinking it solely for the taste, what's the difference?" I was trying to prompt her curiosity about the story she had created that she drank beer solely for the taste.

Let's say you have the option of drinking a Diet Coke or a Coke Zero; one ruins your sleep, makes you send text messages you later regret sending, and causes you to wake up filled with hangxiety, and the other one doesn't affect you at all. Which one would you choose? Probably the one that didn't make you feel awful the next day. So by the same reasoning, if you believe you are drinking alcohol for the taste, why not drink something that doesn't compromise your physical and mental health in the way that alcohol does?

I speak to many women who come to me with similar stories about loving the taste of a glass of wine, whether it's a cold glass of rosé on a summer's day or deep-bodied red with a steak; they love the taste. I can fully relate. Amber, a client who said champagne was her favorite drink in the world, said she loved the flavor of it. She had a few weeks of being alcohol-free under her belt and hopped on a coaching call with me one February day and said, "So, we went out for Valentine's Day."

"Awesome, how'd it go?" I asked.

She explained that she and her date had gone to their special, go-to restaurant, and she had ordered a glass of her favorite champagne. "The taste . . . I don't know. It wasn't the same. I realized it doesn't make me feel good. I couldn't finish the glass."

Another client, Emily, was at a Christmas party a month or so into our coaching. "I can't believe it," she said. "I was handed a beautiful glass of red wine, my favorite, and I couldn't even stomach the idea of drinking it."

Amber and Emily had taken some time off drinking and looked closely at the story "I like to drink because of the taste." Without constant exposure to drinking, their taste buds started to change. They were also armed with the truth about how alcohol was making them feel, and so drinking solely for the taste didn't make sense for them anymore.

We've seen how conditioning and societal influences can sway our preferences and tastes over time. Just as our palates adjust to savor alcohol, they can equally adapt to reject it. Your palate, like your perspective on alcohol, can change, and when it does, there is a world of delightful alcohol-free options waiting to be explored.

As we talked about on day twelve, replacing your nightly cocktail with a mocktail can be helpful when interrupting our habit loops and trying to create new neural pathways. Thankfully, we are spoiled with choices now. If you don't love the idea of replacing your nightly alcoholic drink with a nonalcoholic substitute, experiment with different teas, juices, and smoothies. My "pink lady" of ginger ale, cranberry, and lime did the trick for me. It doesn't necessarily even matter what is in the glass; often, the important part is that it is something that tastes good and feels like a ritual of marking the end of the day with a nice treat.

TiNA

WHAT HAS BEEN YOUR EXPERIENCE WITH THE TASTE of alcohol? Let's get curious. Open your journal and think about the following questions.

1. Did you always like the taste of alcohol? What was your reaction when you first tried it?
2. When did you first enjoy the taste of alcohol? What factors conditioned your sense of taste?
3. Reread today's verses. Who is the one that satisfies our desires with good things?
4. Lastly, make a list of the nonalcoholic drinks that you really enjoy. When you want something delicious to drink, you'll know you have options.

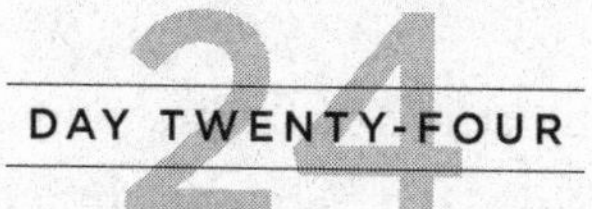

DAY TWENTY-FOUR

The Joy in Leading by Example

He brought them out of darkness, the utter
darkness,
and broke away their chains.

—PSALM 107:14

I ATTENDED A DINNER PARTY ONE EVENING, EXPECTING TO be the only one not drinking. By this point, I was entirely comfortable with my decision to stay sober, but part of me wondered if I would be the odd woman out forever. Just then, one of my girlfriends walked in with a nonalcoholic spirit and asked whether I had any soda water to mix it with. Later in the evening, she said, "Yeah, I quit too. I realize I feel so much better without it."

I was shocked. "Why didn't you tell me?"

"I didn't want it to be a big deal," she said.

After that evening, I had more and more friends ask me about my decision not to drink, and of course, I've had strangers (who have become friends) all over the world ask me via Instagram about this journey. I call this the ripple effect, and I've now seen it happen more times than I can count. My client Megan said, "Being open about my journey has affected others. I think my family members were influenced the most. We have generations of family members who have battled alcohol addiction, and I am changing the cycle."

On day two, I laid out how the cultural drinking landscape is changing for the better, but that might feel very untrue to you if you're the only one you know who is questioning your relationship with alcohol. So, let me encourage you today, my friend. Others will follow you if you're brave enough to start questioning this norm. (And I know you're brave enough.) It might not be immediate, and it might not look like people quitting drinking altogether; I have several friends who drink a lot less than they used to, especially now that I am not ordering another round. You can be the change maker in your group of friends. You can be the leader.

BREAKING THE CYCLE

I wasn't close to my grandfather at all. I only met him in person twice, both times when I was little. He had bipolar disorder and lived in the middle of nowhere on a ranch in Idaho. He verbally and physically abused my mom, although I never knew the true extent. Then, in July 2010, he took his own life. I was in Los Angeles with Ella, who was six months old, when my mom got the call. I watched her break down and quickly turn to alcohol to numb. Her drinking worsened from that point on, and it slowly chipped away at the mother-daughter bond I cherished so deeply.

My mom blamed herself for my grandfather's suicide. The grief compounded with guilt, and the wine exacerbated it all. When my mom drank, she blamed her pain on me and would say I'd abandoned her to move to London and how cruel I was to keep her grandchildren from her. She asked why I had married someone who wanted to live so far away from family. So when she died, I blamed myself. I thought how maybe she wouldn't have been so unhappy and drunk so much if I had been around more.

Then, one day, I got a text from my brother David. "Don't do what she did with her dad. You can't do that. You can't blame yourself." I didn't see it at the time, but he was right. If my children continued to see me drinking to deal with my grief, it would be the only coping mechanism that they understood. I had to do better for them. I had to break the cycle.

When I coach women with a history of alcohol use disorder in their families, they generally tell me, "I come from a long line of alcoholics, which is why my struggle is extra hard." If you relate to this, I have two questions for you:

1. Who would you be without the thought that you're somehow destined to struggle forever because of genetics?
2. What would it feel like to be free of this generational trap?

You can be the change maker in your family and friendships. The fact that you've picked up this book and are getting curious about your journey with alcohol means you're already on your way.

I am now determined that my children have a different understanding of alcohol than I had. One day early on in my journey we were out to lunch as a family. My son, Carter, picked up the wine list and said, "You can't have this, Mommy." I thought for a minute, then replied, "Actually, I can have all the wine I want. I *choose* not to drink it because I don't like how it makes me feel, and I now know how bad it is for me."

Not only have I broken the cycle of drinking by God's grace, but I am proud that I now have the opportunity to teach my children the most meaningful lesson—that we can do hard things with the help of Jesus. I can tell them how alcohol is highly addictive and how Christ helped me overcome it when I started to question the stories I'd believed about alcohol. They get to make their own conscious, empowered choice, armed with some truth.

As you continue on this transformative journey, remember that you get to lead by example. You have the ability to change the trajectory of how your family and friends, your children, your grandchildren, use alcohol. Your bravery in choosing a healthier path can inspire not only those living in your home but also the people all around you and generations to come.

TiNA

TODAY'S TINA MAY SEEM SCARY, BUT I WANT YOU TO do your best not to skip this one. Share with a trusted friend or family member that you are doing this alcohol fast. Remember that talking about it may not feel easy at first, but it might be one of the most important conversations you ever have.

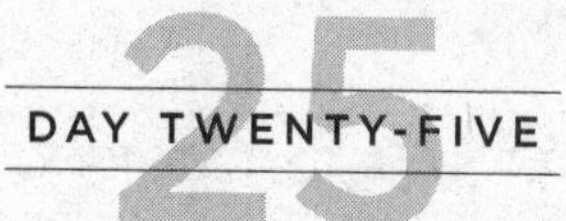

DAY TWENTY-FIVE

Jesus and Wine

"I have the right to do anything," you say—but not everything is beneficial. "I have the right to do anything"—but not everything is constructive.

—1 CORINTHIANS 10:23

I WAS AT LUNCH AT A RESTAURANT IN CHELSEA WITH A BUNCH of girls from Bible study. I was newly sober, and as one of the women ordered a bottle of rosé, she announced, "Well, Jesus drank wine . . . we might as well, right?" It wasn't the first time I had heard this. One of the stories I told myself when I was drinking too much was, *Well, it's okay because Jesus drank wine,* or *Jesus turned water into wine.* I heard it so often that it became the title of my podcast, *"But Jesus Drank Wine" & Other Stories That Kept Us Stuck,* a show where my friend Meade Shirley and I encourage Christian women to find freedom from modern-day drinking culture.

What the Bible says about wine and Jesus's warnings against drunkenness shifted my perspective on my "*but Jesus drank wine*" narrative. Today, let's peel back the layers of this story.

DID JESUS DRINK WINE?

The simple answer is yes. We know that Jesus turned water into wine at the wedding feast at Cana (John 2:1–12) and drank wine with His disciples at the Last Supper (Luke 22:7–38). But there's no evidence that Jesus was ever drunk. The Bible is full of cautionary tales about becoming intoxicated. The apostle Paul warns us with a clear and direct message: "Neither the sexually immoral . . . nor drunkards . . . will inherit the kingdom of God" (1 Corinthians 6:9–10). Peter says that godless people enjoy "drunkenness and wild parties" (1 Peter 4:3, NLT). There isn't one place in the Bible where being intoxicated is portrayed in a positive light, and Paul directly calls it a sin when writing to the early church in Galatia (Galatians 5:19–21).

Now you may be thinking, *Right, I got it. Drunkenness is a sin. But what's wrong with moderation?* As our verse for the day says, we all have the freedom to make choices, but these choices become an issue when they enslave us. Navigating this gray area involves exploring God's Word, understanding our subconscious beliefs, seeking guidance, and prioritizing our desire to be like Christ.

BIBLICAL WINE VS. MODERN-DAY WINE

Jesus was a member of a community that drank wine, and yet He never sinned. He never abused it, let it control Him, or relied upon it. He never used it to relax, cope, or make Himself more joyful. Furthermore, the wine of biblical times was far less addictive because it had a significantly lower alcohol content than contemporary wines. The ancient fermentation processes did not involve the techniques used today. With naturally occurring yeast alone, wine could only reach up to 4 percent alcohol.[1] The introduction of modern-day fermentation methods occurred in the thirteenth century, allowing today's wines to have an alcohol by volume (ABV) as high as 14.5 percent.[2] Consequently, the alcohol Jesus drank at Passover contained much less alcohol than the wine readily available to us today.[3]

Unlike in biblical times, when fermented drinks required time to produce and were not easily accessible, today we have a ready supply of alcohol, which can even be delivered to our doorstep. I once coached a client who during the Covid lockdown felt trapped at home with nothing to do and consequently developed a habit of ordering cases of wine. Many clients have shared similar stories of having alcohol delivered regularly. We must acknowledge that we are dealing with a vastly different cultural landscape than in the biblical era, where alcoholic drinks were not as readily available as they are today.

IS ALCOHOL AN IDOL?

God commands in Exodus, "You shall have no other gods before me."[4] At first glance, it may not seem like alcohol qualifies as an idol—after all, we're not worshipping wine bottles. But upon closer examination of why I drank, how I drank, and how much I was relying on my drinking, the truth became apparent. I had turned to alcohol to fulfill roles in my life—such as expecting it to bring me joy and heal me from grief—that only God could truly fulfill. Additionally, the significant amount of time, money, and mental energy I dedicated to wine had unquestionably elevated it to the status of an idol in my life.

But how are we to know when our drinking has crossed over into becoming an idol? Jesus said in Matthew 6:24, "No one can serve two masters. Either you will hate the one and love the other, or you will be devoted to the one and despise the other. You cannot serve both God and money." What if we swapped out the word *money* for *wine* in that sentence? Does it hit home for you as it did for me?

Idols have a cunning way of making us believe they bring comfort, all the while keeping us disconnected from the Comforter. Paul said in 2 Corinthians 1:3–5, "Praise be to the God and Father of our Lord Jesus Christ, the Father of compassion and the God of all comfort, who comforts us in all our troubles, so that we can comfort those in any trouble with the comfort we ourselves receive from God. For just as we share abundantly in the sufferings of Christ, so also our comfort abounds through Christ."

Alcohol deceived me into thinking it provided comfort, which led me to rely on drinking instead of seeking comfort in Christ. This is how alcohol became an idol for me—it lied and disconnected me from God.

So let me encourage you today, my beautiful friend; God is the ultimate source of true peace, rest, hope, and comfort. Alcohol merely serves as an inadequate substitute.

TiNA

In what ways have you justified your drinking patterns over the years? Take a minute to pray—as honestly as you can—about your worries, struggles, and thoughts about alcohol. Ask God to journey with you as your help and guide.

Recall moments when you felt a deep sense of God's peace and comfort in your life. How can you intentionally nurture your connection with and reliance on the Comforter instead of seeking comfort in alcohol? By reading the Word? By spending time in prayer? Through connecting with other Christians? Write down your intentions.

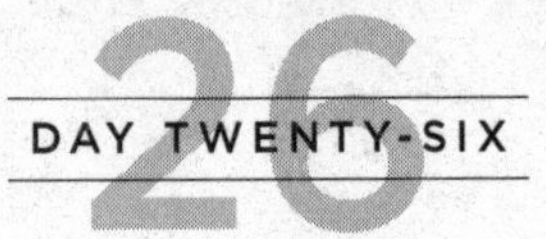

DAY TWENTY-SIX

The Science of Joy

Always be full of joy in the Lord.
I say it again—rejoice!

—PHILIPPIANS 4:4, NLT

I OFTEN ASK MY CLIENTS IF THERE WAS A *WOW* MOMENT WHEN they felt their joy come back online after decades of drinking.

Sarah in Texas said, "Swimming in the ocean completely sober for the first time in years was the moment for me. Most beach vacations in my twenties started with drinks in the morning, so jumping in the waves sober brought back childhood happiness and joy that I hadn't felt in years."

Amelia in Massachusetts had this to say about her *wow* moment, "I took a sober trip to our lake house for the first time in probably twenty years. I grew up going up there every weekend and had completely lost perspective on how much I love it up there. This summer, during a walk, I felt refreshed, relaxed, awake, grateful, and happy to be taking in the beautiful views. I realized the happiness I was feeling was possible because the alcohol was out of my system. My feelings had returned!"

I once believed that alcohol brought me joy. So when I looked back at my photo reel to pictures of me holding a glass of wine at a fancy restaurant or sipping a margarita at the beach, I equated those times with happiness. And sure, I may have felt happy at the beginning of a night of drinking. But it never ended that way.

I had lots of little *wow* moments as I felt my joy return in the early days of sobriety. I walked in the park and saw the sun sparkle on the river Thames and thanked God I had the opportunity to live in my favorite city in the world. I snuggled on the couch with Chris and the kids to watch a family movie and eat popcorn and felt overwhelming joy and contentment. I laughed hysterically in the kitchen as my then tween daughter taught me silly TikTok dances. I remember the thrill and excitement from my children when I actually got in the ocean with them on vacation instead of staying on my lounger to drink rosé.

It was utterly fascinating to me when I learned the neurochemistry of how alcohol was zapping my joy. But when I *felt* the difference, I was convinced that the science was spot-on.

DOPAMINE'S EVIL COUSIN, DYNORPHIN

On day five, we talked about how our brain reacts when we drink alcohol. We know that drinking provides a temporary euphoria, driven by a dopamine and endorphin release in our brains. However, this rush is artificial and overrides our bodies' natural production of these pleasure hormones. In response, our brains release a counteracting chemical called dynorphin, a "buzzkill" hormone, to restore balance. Instead of appreciating this rebalancing act, we often chase the initial high from the first drink, though it's scientifically impossible to replicate. Each subsequent sip doesn't make us happier; rather, it numbs us and fills us with a depressant that takes days to wear off.[1] Thus, alcohol, while momentarily uplifting, ultimately brings us down. Think about this for a second: Do you usually wake up feeling happy and energized after a night of drinking?

Our brains link not only the act of drinking alcohol with a dopamine rush but everything associated with it—walking in the door at the end of the day, getting out the wine glass, or sitting in your usual drinking spot. Our brains know a dopamine hit is coming. So what do they do? They release dynorphin in anticipation of getting that feel-good rush. Hence, when you're a regular drinker, you're pumping yourself with a depressant sedative before you even start drinking.[2]

Over time, the brain gets so used to receiving this massive injection of dopamine all the time that it stops producing so much of it, and slowly, we erase our natural production of this essential neurochemical.[3] What does this look like? It means eventually you're unable to experience joy unless you're drinking. It means you're unable to laugh with friends without a glass of wine in your hand. This means you're unable to feel joy when you're watching your son's soccer game or your daughter's dance recital. It means you're unable to stop to appreciate God's blessings around you because you can't feel happy without alcohol. When you're building up a tolerance to alcohol, you also build up a tolerance to joy and happiness.

When I realized that I had been pumping myself full of a chemical that killed my joy, it hit me hard. I had missed so much joy and laughter with my family. How could I have dulled so many happy memories with my children? I was shocked, but it also made so much sense because when I stopped drinking, I felt my joy return.

Joy is a fruit of the Spirit; it's supposed to shine in us so brightly as believers that others know we are Christ followers. Our joy is in Christ Jesus, who died and saved us and loves us for eternity. As a drinker, I was not living my life rooted in this joy. I was sad, grumpy, and irritable all the time. As the ancient proverb says, "A joyful heart is good medicine, but a crushed spirit dries up the bones" (Proverbs 17:22, ESV).

You may have heard of the pink cloud effect when you take a break from alcohol. This is where everything around you feels happy and wonderful because your regular dopamine production is returning. The chemicals that made you feel down in the dumps are clearing out of your system. Many people say this pink cloud effect fades, but I don't believe this is true for Christians. When we are reconnected with Jesus and the joy of living our lives for Him, this fruit of the Spirit is here to stay.

TiNA

THINK ABOUT MOMENTS IN YOUR LIFE WHEN YOU experienced genuine joy and happiness without the influence of alcohol. Write down these moments and describe what made them special. How did they make you feel, and what aspects of those moments can you incorporate into your life to bring back that pure joy? How have you noticed your joy returning, in big or small ways? How does the reminder that Jesus is our joy shift your thoughts and assumptions about drinking? What feelings seem to be awakening for you, and which ones are you still waiting for?

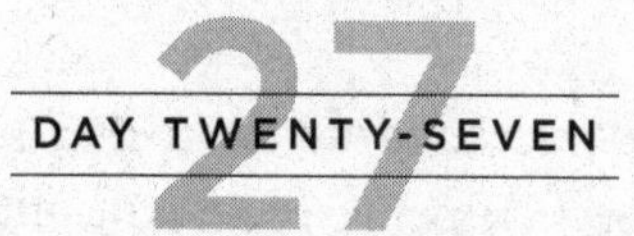

DAY TWENTY-SEVEN

Alcohol and Anxiety

God has not given us a spirit of fear, but of power and of love and of sound mind.

—2 TIMOTHY 1:7, NKJV

MY STOMACH WAS CHURNING, MY BODY FELT SHAKY, the anxiety was overwhelming. I sat down to complete my first morning session of the three-day California bar exam in a massive ballroom in the basement of a Los Angeles hotel. I had hired tutors and studied the entire summer before the exam, and I was determined, despite it being known as the most challenging bar exam in the US, to pass it on my first go-around. I fired up my laptop, made nervous small talk with my deskmate, and waited for the proctor to say, "Begin."

I dove into the first essay question and started outlining my answer. About twenty minutes into the most important exam of my life, the massive ballroom chandeliers began to tremble. It was an earthquake. I watched as dozens of recent law graduates decided to ditch the test and run for safety. I noticed my deskmate wasn't moving. *Am I going to die during an earthquake during the California bar exam? What a way to go.*

I made the split-second decision that I had worked too hard to run out on this exam. I had vowed I would only take this test once, and no earthquake would get in the way of that. I stayed and furiously typed despite the shaking. The proctor never stopped the test. The morning session ended. Then came the afternoon session. And then, finally, day one was done. I still had two days left to go, but the shock and stress of that quaky morning led me to order a bottle of wine the second I returned to my hotel room. I poured a massive glass of red and then a second, as was my practice after finishing any stressful exam. I thought the wine would ease my anxiety, calm me down, and help me get through anything I was nervous about.

Everything I'd ever seen or heard told me alcohol was the key to de-stressing. I had no idea my drinking was making my stress even more unmanageable.

ALCOHOL INCREASES OUR STRESS

Sure, that first sip of alcohol might give you a fleeting sense of euphoria, but what follows is a surge in cortisol, the body's stress hormone.[1] It's like pouring gasoline on the stress fire. Each sip of alcohol boosts the body's baseline cortisol production, creating a continuous state of heightened anxiety, particularly for regular drinkers. I remember feeling constantly stressed and on edge when I was drinking. Research shows that alcohol increases cortisol levels not only while drinking but also for some time afterward, during withdrawal, contributing to a cycle of chronic stress levels.[2]

It Doesn't Help the Root of the Problem

Drinking can distract us from the stresses we're facing, but the situation we're working to de-stress from is usually still there in the morning. Drinking never fixes the root of the anxiety-causing problem. Whether we're drinking because we're anxious about our marriage, our job, our children, an exam, or our financial situation, alcohol doesn't help with any of it. The issue remains, and now we've added a hangover, lousy sleep, and heightened cortisol on top of it.

It Ruins Your Sleep

If you've ever fallen asleep with a glass of wine on your bedside table, you know how quickly alcohol can make you feel sleepy. But as we learned on day sixteen, alcohol hijacks our REM sleep. If you're a regular drinker, you're likely living in perpetual exhaustion. Additionally, because of the way alcohol dehydrates us and throws off our hormones, we end up waking up in the night, often with zero ability to fall back asleep. Lack of sleep is a surefire way to make any tense situation more challenging.

Alcohol Impairs Judgment

My client Lacey described alcohol as the "mental sledgehammer" she used to stop all the noise her anxiety would cause. However, when she took a break from drinking, she realized how quickly that sledgehammer effect wore off and how it often made things much worse. Alcohol had given her a few minutes of relief but came with massive consequences, and she decided the trade-off wasn't worth it.

When we drink to quiet our minds, we slow down our prefrontal cortex—the decision-making part of our brain responsible for planning and impulse control. It can also dampen our ability to properly assess risks,[3] leading us to do things we wouldn't do sober. These natural effects of alcohol can leave us more stressed out than when we started.

Ever had that sinking feeling the morning after a night of drinking that has you scared to check your phone for fear of whom or what you may have texted? Or maybe you cringe at a memory of something you did or said while buzzed? That's hangxiety—a cocktail of regret and anxiety stirred up by alcohol. And what do we often do when this feeling becomes overwhelming and we need to escape it? More booze. When we drink to manage our anxiety, we lose perspective of this quick-fix–horrible-consequences-later cycle.

GIVING POWER TO ANXIETY

When we drink, we're often unintentionally giving power to the source of our anxiety and frustration. My client Megan in New York City drank primarily for one reason: the state of America. Post-Covid health policies, immigration legislation, school shootings, and pretty much everything else she watched on the news made her anxious. Her solution was to drown out the state of the world with wine. Then one day as we were chatting in a coaching session, I said, "Megan, do you realize that drinking to deal with the stress of political unrest is handing all your power to those politicians you keep telling me you dislike?" She looked at me, shocked.

We worked on how we could change her thinking about her worries and anxieties and use better coping mechanisms (such as turning off the news and staying off Facebook), and these practices helped her not to reach for the wine bottle every time a news alert popped up on her phone.

For Megan to get her anxiety under control, she had to figure out precisely what was stirring up her anxious thoughts in the first place and determine if focusing on those things, which she had no control over, was serving her.

Does this mean that our stress will completely vanish without alcohol? Not necessarily. Life's stressors continue to exist, but without alcohol, you're better equipped to handle them. You place yourself in a much better position when your hormones, including adrenaline and cortisol, are in balance, when you're well rested and clearheaded, and when you have the ability to take your anxious thoughts captive.

We are fighting a battle in our minds, whether we're clouding it with alcohol or not. The Enemy is there, planning and planting those negative thoughts day in and day out, hoping we grab on to them and spiral into anxiety. But we have the ability to check our anxious thoughts against the truth. The truth is that God is in control, and we are not. He knows the number of hairs on our heads and always knows His plans for us.[4]

The following are a few quotes from clients about how drinking affected their anxiety:

My strongest belief was that alcohol helped me relax and relieve stress. However, when I really thought about it and examined my nightly wine ritual and the path it led me down, there was nothing relaxing about it. It was just the opposite and caused sleepless nights and hangxiety.

—Kimberly

Hangover anxiety was the worst. And the older I got, the harder it hit. To "calm" my hangover anxiety from the weekend, I would drink again on Sundays, but then I was a mess of worry and sadness until Wednesday at least. I had to offer so many next-day apologies. My anxiety decreased immediately after I stopped drinking.

—Michelle

My strongest belief was that alcohol helped with my anxiety. But my anxiety was so crippling after drinking that I knew alcohol must be causing massive pain instead of relieving it. My most anxious thoughts usually started at four in the morning, and they were on overdrive. The guilt, shame, and insecurity would come crashing in. I learned that alcohol soothed anxiety for the first thirty minutes after drinking, but the aftermath is what creates the ongoing cycle. Now that I am not drinking, I only really experience situational anxiety, which I can overcome with healthy tools.

—Amy

TiNA

THE NEXT TIME YOU BEGIN TO FEEL ANXIOUS ABOUT something, try to take the thoughts captive. Write them down. What story are you telling yourself, and is it true? I know that when we're in the throes of an anxious mind-swirl, this can feel really hard. But remember to run the anxious thoughts through the truth of God's Word. Matthew 6:27–34 is a great place to start:

> Can any one of you by worrying add a single hour to your life?
>
> And why do you worry about clothes? See how the flowers of the field grow. They do not labor or spin. Yet I tell you that not even Solomon in all his splendor was dressed like one of these. If that is how God clothes the grass of the field, which is here today and tomorrow is thrown into the fire, will he not much more clothe you—you of little faith? So do not worry, saying, "What shall we eat?" or "What shall we drink?" or "What shall we wear?" For the pagans run after all these things, and your heavenly Father knows that you need them. But seek first his kingdom and his righteousness, and all these things will be given to you as well. Therefore do not worry about tomorrow, for tomorrow will worry about itself. Each day has enough trouble of its own.

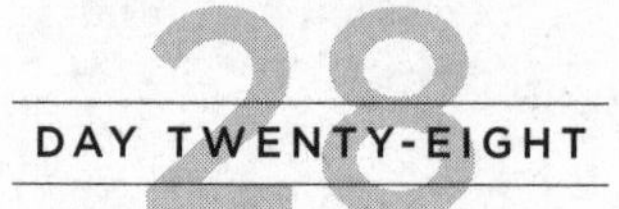

DAY TWENTY-EIGHT

Renewing Your Confidence

But those who hope in the Lord
will renew their strength.
They will soar on wings like eagles;
they will run and not grow weary,
they will walk and not be faint.

—ISAIAH 40:31

When I sat down for my first session with Grace, a mom of three from London, we began chatting about why she wanted to take a break from alcohol. "I want to get my confidence back," she said. However, when we moved into discussing her stories about alcohol, they were deeply rooted in the assumption that without liquid courage, she didn't know how to socialize. I could relate to Grace's story because I had also relied on cocktails to make me a better party companion.

Let's investigate this assumption with our Awareness → Story → Truth tactic we learned on day eight.

1. Identify the thought. What job are you giving alcohol, or why do you think you like to drink it? In Grace's case, it might be something like this: *Drinking makes me more confident.*

2. Investigate the story. Where did this belief come from? What are the facts, and what story are you using to fill in the gaps? For example, perhaps it's been a long time since you've been to a social gathering where you haven't drunk, so your brain seems to have evidence that without alcohol you can't socialize.
3. What's the truth? Let's dive deeper to find out.

THE CONFIDENCE KILLER

When we take those first few sips of alcohol and the edge comes off, we feel like we can more easily talk to others. Our prefrontal cortex (the decision-making part of our brains) is slowly going offline, so naturally our inhibitions lower and we feel less nervous. For some reason, we focus on this part of the evening instead of what happens next. After a few drinks, we may lose focus on the conversation and wind up chatting with strangers or broaching sensitive subjects we know we shouldn't. Have you ever woken up the morning after a night out feeling regret over spilling your deepest, darkest secrets or gossiping about someone you care about? I sure have. Lowered inhibitions coupled with hangxiety silently destroy our self-confidence and leave us second-guessing our actions, doubting our self-worth, and undermining the very confidence that we sought alcohol to boost in the first place.

THE BROKEN PROMISES

Before I quit drinking for good, I made a lot of attempts at moderation. Moderation for me meant laying down tons of ground rules only for those rules to be inevitably broken over the course of the evening. And because I repeatedly couldn't keep my word, thanks to alcohol's addictive nature, I lost faith in myself.

I've spoken with many women who feel shame and regret over not being able to stick to their moderation rules. They feel like if they can't just have one or two drinks, something must be wrong with them. Playing a losing game of moderation over and over can erode your confidence. But remember, God didn't make you the one woman on the planet who can't moderate her wine. Anyone can get addicted to an addictive substance.

THE REAL DEAL ABOUT CONFIDENCE

Confidence is often misunderstood as something innate or naturally occurring within us. In reality, it is neither. True confidence emerges as a result of taking action and acquiring competence. It doesn't simply appear on its own; it requires stepping out of your comfort zone and embracing challenges. You must be willing to try and tackle the difficult tasks to nurture and grow your confidence. I often ask clients, "Do you want to be comfortable, or do you want to grow?"

Grace and I started working together at the beginning of December, so the season's holiday parties gave her plenty of opportunities to get more confident. She began going to those parties and turning down the champagne. She said the first fifteen minutes were awkward, but she soon found her stride. I'll never forget when she popped on a call with me and exclaimed, "I think I found my confidence, and I didn't even need a drink!"

VISUALIZATION

I often give my clients the following tactic when they are feeling insecure about not drinking in social situations.

Pick one trusted friend, maybe it's your best friend or your spouse, and make a plan to go out to dinner. Recognize the moments you are nervous about and visualize a specific plan for how you want to handle them before you go out for the meal.

For example, are you nervous about ordering a nonalcoholic drink? Pick one ahead of time and have the answer ready. Are you worried about what you will chat about with your friend? Think about a few topics to get the conversation started. Get as specific as you can about what's holding you back.

Michael Phelps, the greatest swimmer of our time, is known for using visualization techniques to win Olympic gold medals. "I would visualize the best- and worst-case scenarios. Whether I get disqualified, or my goggles fill up with water, or I lose my goggles, or I come in last, I'm ready for anything," he said.[1] We can use the same tactic when helping grow our confidence in sobriety.

The next time you're worried about not having confidence without alcohol, plan for every variable. Visualize the entire meal or evening. Be ready for anything. I promise you that it gets easier. It just takes practice.

WE WILL NOT FEAR

Remember this incredibly good news: When we don't feel confident, we can call on Jesus for help. We have an ever-present source of strength and guidance in Jesus Christ. Here are a few reminders of His unwavering support:

- "God is our refuge and strength, an ever-present help in trouble. Therefore we will not fear, though the earth give way and the mountains fall into the heart of the sea" (Psalm 46:1–2).
- "Let us then approach God's throne of grace with confidence, so that we may receive mercy and find grace to help us in our time of need" (Hebrews 4:16).
- "Cast all your anxiety on him because he cares for you" (1 Peter 5:7).
- "Be strong and courageous. Do not be afraid or terrified because of them, for the LORD your God goes with you; he will never leave you nor forsake you" (Deuteronomy 31:6).
- " 'For I know the plans I have for you,' declares the LORD, 'plans to prosper you and not to harm you, plans to give you hope and a future' " (Jeremiah 29:11).

Lean on Jesus. Hold His promises close to your heart. He is always ready to assist you on your journey.

I examined my belief that alcohol made me more confident, and after considering the truth, here's where I landed: Alcohol actually eroded my confidence. But here I am now, alcohol-free and more confident than I have ever been. I know my value in Christ Jesus as one of His daughters.

I recently checked in with Grace. "Do you feel more self-confident?"

"One thousand percent!" she said. "I'm so proud of myself, and I feel strong."

If Grace and I can rediscover our confidence, you will too.

TiNA

VISUALIZE YOUR NEXT SOCIAL OUTING. CONSIDER the best-case and worst-case scenarios. What simple steps can you do to prepare yourself ahead of time, like reviewing menus online or determining what time you plan to be home?

When you do attend an event, pay close attention to how long any social awkwardness lasts. Push through that uncomfortable feeling and notice that it is temporary.

As you end this TiNA, talk to God about what still feels hard and celebrate what is starting to feel more manageable.

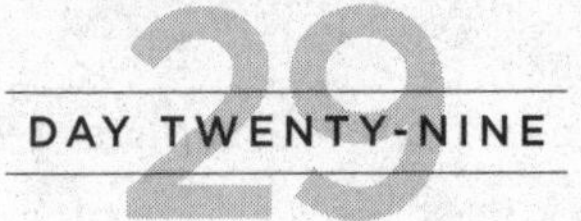

DAY TWENTY-NINE

The Hidden Dangers of Alcohol

Do not gaze at wine when it is red,
when it sparkles in the cup,
when it goes down smoothly!
In the end it bites like a snake
and poisons like a viper.

—PROVERBS 23:31–32

BEFORE I QUIT DRINKING, I WAS VERY CONCERNED ABOUT everything *besides* the wine I was putting in my body. I researched the differences between coconut, soy, almond, and oat milk to ensure I chose the healthiest one. I spent a fortune on green smoothies and green juices. But I never stopped to think about what was in my wine glass.

I will never forget the time I was researching the health risks of alcohol and came across the chemical compound of alcohol. Alcohol contains ethanol, the same chemical composition as the ethanol in gasoline, which we fill our cars with.[1] Can you imagine guzzling down gas from the nozzle at a gas station? That would be bizarre and gross.

Once you sip your cocktail, the body recognizes the alcohol as a toxin and quickly goes to work, trying to break it down and get rid of it as fast as possible. Anything else that needs to be digested gets put on the back burner, so your digestion immediately slows down. After the alcohol travels through your bloodstream, through the lining of your stomach and small intestine, it arrives at the liver, where enzymes convert the alcohol into a class 1 carcinogen known as acetaldehyde.[2] This toxic compound is very harmful to our bodies and increases our cancer risk. You know what else is classified as a class 1 carcinogen? Tobacco, asbestos, formaldehyde, and plutonium.[3] And yet, at the time of writing this book we don't have adequate warning labels on alcohol.

The harm alcohol wreaks on our health is very real and far more significant than I first realized. The purpose of today's chapter is not to scare you but to empower you with information on how alcohol is affecting your health.

THE LIVER

Let's start with the most obvious victim, the liver. The liver is responsible for breaking down and removing toxins from our body, and drinking can lead to liver damage, including fatty liver disease, cirrhosis, and hepatitis. I used to believe this only happened to older men who drank a lot of hard liquor; but the fact is, there is a massive spike in women, and young women, struggling with liver problems. Dr. James Burton, medical director of liver transplantation at the University of Colorado School of Medicine in Aurora, points out the increase in young women with liver disease needing a transplant has skyrocketed in the last few years because of the increase in their drinking. "Last year, I took care of two women who were in their early 20s who had cirrhosis and needed liver transplants, and I've never seen that before in my entire career," he says.[4] A startling surge in alcohol-related liver disease has been observed recently, leading to a 15 percent rise in the number of patients on waiting lists for liver transplants, notably from overuse during the pandemic years of 2020 and 2021. Alarmingly, young adults are experiencing the most substantial increase in these cases.[5]

A 2024 study forecasts that healthcare-related expenditures on women dealing with alcohol-related liver diseases are expected to soar, with costs for women making up 43 percent of the total annual expenditure by 2040, up from 29 percent in 2022.[6] This represents a drastic spike in healthcare spending for women, underscoring a crisis that can no longer be ignored.

I'll never forget Karla Adkins, who graciously shared her story on my podcast. Through tears she explained how she looked in the mirror one day and saw that her eyes had turned yellow. She was only thirty-seven years old and was diagnosed with acute liver failure. Karla now shares her story of recovering from the disease in the hopes that other women don't have to make the same phone call she did. "I'm dying," she said to her father.

"Well, I want you to focus on living," he replied.[7]

Here's some incredible news for you: Liver specialists have discovered the remarkable regenerative capacity of this vital organ. Studies have shown that just a few weeks of abstinence from alcohol can have a monumental effect on liver regeneration. The longer you stay alcohol-free, the greater the chance of healing for your liver.[8]

THE HEART

I grew up with the story that red wine was good for my heart. Did you? Big alcohol used to love to cite research that resveratrol, found in red wine from the skin of the grapes, was good for your heart health. This is because of its links to lowering cholesterol and preventing blood clots. However, *new* science (not funded by big alcohol) says that the amount of resveratrol in red wine isn't enough to have preventative effects.[9] Big alcohol found *one* decent ingredient in red wine and claimed the whole glass was good for you.

In 2021, the World Heart Federation released a report to ensure this old study was put to bed. "The evidence is clear: Any level of alcohol consumption can lead to the loss of healthy life. Studies have shown that even small amounts of alcohol can increase a person's risk of cardiovascular disease, including coronary disease, stroke, heart failure, hypertensive heart disease, and aneurysm."[10] Drinking alcohol can cause irregular heartbeats and lead to cardiomyopathy, a condition in which the heart muscle becomes damaged.[11] In addition, the American College of Cardiology states that even moderate alcohol consumption can increase the risk of atrial fibrillation, a dangerous type of irregular heartbeat.[12]

CANCER

Reducing our alcohol consumption opens up a world of transformative health benefits, and one of the most significant is a lowered risk of at least six types of cancer, including mouth, throat, esophagus, liver, breast, and colon cancer.[13]

Most women don't know that just three alcoholic drinks per week gives them a 15 percent higher risk of breast cancer compared to those who abstain. Moreover, each additional daily drink increases that risk by another 10 percent.[14] Three drinks per week? I was usually having three drinks per day.

According to Cancer Research UK, approximately one in ten breast cancer diagnoses are linked to alcohol consumption.[15] Notably, the risk of developing breast cancer escalates even with low levels of alcohol intake.

GUT HEALTH

Your gut health is the unsung hero of your body's well-being, cultivating a remarkable ecosystem of good bacteria crucial to your health. It's a key player in digestion, metabolism, and your immune response. Think of this complex microbiome as an internal garden that thrives when well nourished and cared for. When you opt out of drinking alcohol, you're giving this garden the chance to flourish.

Alcohol can disrupt this delicate balance with bloating, constipation, and diarrhea. It may also lead to acid reflux and other gastrointestinal issues.[16] Multiple clients have shared with me that they had spent years suffering with IBS but the minute they stopped drinking, their stomach issues resolved.

But the benefits don't stop there. Your gut is intricately linked to your brain and helps regulate your mood, appetite, and sleep.[17] By saying no to alcohol, you're not just nurturing your physical health but also safeguarding your mental health.

HERE'S TO YOUR HEALTH

Every time you chose not to pick up that drink in the past twenty-nine days and every bottle you left unopened, you've given yourself some of the greatest gifts imaginable: a healthier body and a clearer mind.

Jesus said in John 10:10, "I have come that they may have

life, and have it to the full." So, let's stay curious and keep our focus on living. Armed with truth and with the help of our heavenly Father, we get to make our own conscious, empowered decisions about alcohol and how it affects us living our best lives for Him.

TiNA

REMEMBER, THE PURPOSE OF TODAY'S CHAPTER IS NOT to scare you, but to help empower you. What were the "health benefits" of alcohol that you heard about growing up? Consider what information in today's reading was brand-new or familiar to you. Think about how much time you have spent considering other health topics like gluten, sugar, meat, and dairy. Is it time to give the same consideration to alcohol?

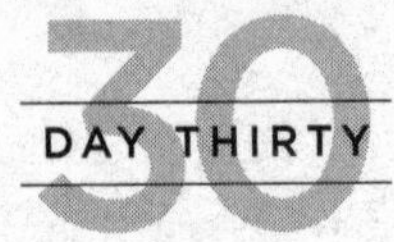

DAY THIRTY

Wellness in Disguise

Trust in the Lord *with all your heart*
and lean not on your own understanding;
in all your ways submit to him,
and he will make your paths straight.

—PROVERBS 3:5–6

There is a new covert alcohol marketing tactic that has become popular as of late: Enter "clean" alcohol. Cameron Diaz recently launched her "clean wine" company called Avaline. The website claims the wine contains "100% organic grapes" with "no added sugar" and "no unwanted additives" and is "vegan."[1] Another brand called "Mom Water" is fruit-flavored vodka. It is marketed as containing zero sugar, zero carbs, and only ninety calories per can. The flavors are even named after real women like "Sandy" and "Linda" and "Julie."[2] Recently, an Instagram ad popped up advertising another similar alcohol brand. The tagline read, "Why choose between taste and health when you can have both?" These brands and their deceptive marketing tactics are aimed right at women who want to make healthier choices. The "organic" and "no additives" language is entirely misleading.

Here's the bottom line. You can take out all the sugar and sulfites, but when grapes are fermented and produce ethanol, the addictive and cancer-causing part of the wine is still present. Ethanol cannot be cleaned. Ethanol causes all the health risks we learned about yesterday.

In a world where we're bombarded with seemingly "healthier" alcoholic products every day, it's essential to recognize that alcohol has long attempted to masquerade as a healthy choice. I've witnessed champagne being offered after Pilates classes and wine tastings at wellness retreats, creating a covert connection between alcohol and well-being. This subtle association between alcohol and health is then stored in our subconscious and leads us to make misinformed choices about alcohol. By staying curious and seeking truth beyond marketing slogans, we can reclaim our autonomy and make choices that genuinely serve our well-being.

PINKWASHING

Anne used to work in marketing for one of the massive alcohol companies and later for a craft brewery company. She and I recently talked about marketing tactics we have seen or used that were specifically aimed at women. When I asked her what key things she sold to women alongside alcohol for effective marketing, she responded, "Fun and connection." And then she explained pinkwashing.

During October, Breast Cancer Awareness Month, alcohol brands "pinkwash" the alcohol bottles, wrapping them up in pretty pink packaging and adding the pink breast cancer awareness ribbon on the liquor bottles or advertisements to "support" women. In one specific campaign Anne herself worked on, the brand offered free drinks at particular bars to women who could show they had a mammogram. We now know that alcohol is one of the leading causes of breast cancer and that even one drink per day can increase your risk.[3] Still, this doesn't stop big alcohol from doing whatever it can to keep women buying drinks.

THE GOOD NEWS

Times are changing. Governments are struggling to justify the health risks and deaths caused each year by alcohol. Canada stepped up in recent years and changed the country's drinking guidelines. The old guidelines allowed a maximum of ten drinks per week for women and fifteen drinks for men. In 2023, they drastically changed the recommendations based on health risks and now advise that citizens avoid alcohol altogether, with the maximum amount recommended being two drinks a week for both men and women.[4]

Ireland is taking the lead in the European Union by adding warning labels on wine, beer, and spirits. The proposed labels will clearly communicate three vital health warnings: Alcohol consumption is a known cause of liver disease, alcohol use is directly linked to life-threatening cancers, and consuming alcohol during pregnancy poses serious risks to the unborn child.[5]

Hopefully, we will get new and improved warning labels in the US and the rest of the world soon. According to the *New England Journal of Medicine,* "Alcohol consumption and its associated harms are reaching a crisis point in the United States. Evidence suggests that new alcohol warnings could empower consumers to make more informed decisions and reduce alcohol-related harm."[6] Currently, the outdated warning labels in the US mainly only cite risks to pregnancy and the risks of operating heavy machinery in tiny text on the backs of the bottles. These labels don't include anything about the risks of cancer, high blood pressure, or liver disease.

TRUST IN THE LORD, NOT IN MARKETING TACTICS

As we unravel the deceptive tactics of alcohol marketing and gain a deeper understanding of its impact on our health, we empower ourselves to make informed choices. The shifting guidelines, the calls for more informative warning labels, and the growing awareness from government agencies are all signs of progress. And together, we can keep educating ourselves, reminding ourselves and the women in our lives what's truly good for us, and championing healthier decisions.

TiNA

HOW HAS ALCOHOL MARKETING INFLUENCED YOUR choice of whether or not to drink? Take a second and do a Google images search; type something like "alcohol pinkwash breast cancer." Knowing what you know now about alcohol's role in causing this deadly disease, how do these images make you feel? Here is the encouraging news: You have a choice to lower your risk of cancer by not drinking. It's an incredible benefit of sobriety that I had no idea about until I did my research. Knowledge is power, babe.

31

DAY THIRTY-ONE

Redefining Fun

Make me walk along the path of your commands,
for that is where my happiness is found.

—PSALM 119:35, NLT

ONE SUMMER DAY, I MET A FRIEND FOR A WALK IN Battersea Park. I was about four months into my sobriety journey, and we ended up talking about my journey. She asked, "But what about the summer? There's no way you can go through the whole summer and trips to the beach without drinking rosé!"

I felt my panic rising because I had the same fear. I thought of a specific day the previous summer. Four of my girlfriends from London had flown to Los Angeles for vacation. We sat at the beach and drank and giggled for hours. My dad and brother turned up. It was warm, the sun was shining, and we watched my children run and play in the ocean. I thought about that day and couldn't imagine it without the rosé, which I believed was fueling the fun. But then I ran that story through the truth. I listed all the things that made that particular day so enjoyable. It was because I had some of my favorite people in my favorite place, with incredible weather.

So why was I giving alcohol all the credit?

I've heard clients say they're worried about life getting boring if they don't drink, and I get that. But now, after years of sobriety, I can tell you that the "fun" I was hanging on to wasn't fun anymore—the late nights, the memory loss, the arguments, the hangovers, the shame. When I stopped drinking, I felt an overwhelming sense of peace, not boredom. I realized I was confusing fun with chaos and boredom with peace.

A NEW KIND OF FUN

I stopped drinking at the time many of my friends were celebrating their fortieth birthdays, and it felt like there was so much pressure to do something big—a big party, a big trip, something over-the-top to mark the milestone. As my fortieth birthday approached, I thought about how I wanted to spend it. I didn't want to simply appease other people or make a big splash on Instagram, but I wanted to celebrate with the people I loved the most. I did a few small get-togethers with girlfriends and then spent three days in the Cotswolds over my birthday weekend with Chris, the kids, and the dog. We watched Christmas movies, snuggled by a fire, and ate cake. It was the perfect birthday. There were no massive parties, no late nights, just sweet memories with the people I loved the most. It was perfect.

If you had told thirty-five-year-old Christy that I would spend my fortieth birthday sitting on the couch in my pajamas, she would have been horrified. But my definition of fun has changed for the better. Yours, if you stay open and curious, can too.

C. S. Lewis wrote, "In commanding us to glorify Him, God invites us to enjoy Him."[1] God wants us to enjoy the blessings He has given us. Now that I am not drinking, I find ordinary things that I used to think were boring are fun: walks with my dog, a great exercise class, a game of padel, and movie nights with the kids. When we're present to it, life is full of little joys.

RETURNING TO OLD LOVES

Sally, from West Palm Beach, Florida, started working with me after decades of drinking. She realized that she had no idea how to have fun unless alcohol was involved. I encouraged her to go back and think about her childhood and what she enjoyed back then. She smiled and said, "I used to be a dancer." I encouraged her to find a few different dance classes in her area, and together we worked on her finding joy in dance again.

One of my favorite parts of this job is helping women reconnect with old loves—the things they delighted in before alcohol crept in and stole the show.

Taking a break from alcohol isn't about misery and missing out, it's about discovering all the things that light you up. It's about enjoying God and His blessings and creation without a class 1 carcinogen dulling your senses and stealing your true joy. It's about reconnecting with who you really are and designing a life that you love.

TiNA

IS THERE AN EVENT OR DAY YOU'RE HOLDING ON TO, like I was, that is contributing to your story that you can't have fun without alcohol? Is it possible you have been giving alcohol more credit than it deserves? Pick up your journal and write about what was truly enjoyable about this experience. What did you love—the company, the weather, the food, the music? What opportunities do you have in your weekly routine to build in more of what you truly enjoy?

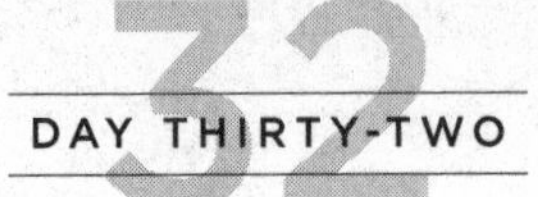

DAY THIRTY-TWO

Filling the Gap and Embracing Our Emotions

Do nothing out of selfish ambition or vain conceit. Rather, in humility value others above yourselves, not looking to your own interests but each of you to the interests of the others.

—PHILIPPIANS 2:3–4

ONE OF MY CLIENTS, VICTORIA, IS MARRIED TO A SUCCESSful lawyer who spends a lot of time in the office. When we sat down for our first session, and I asked her for her list of reasons why she likes to drink, she replied, "I drink to fill the gap." As the wife of a hardworking lawyer who also spent a lot of late nights at the office, I understood what she was saying. There had been many nights over the years when the kids were asleep but Chris was still working and I was alone and bored. A bottle of cabernet filled the gap.

I hear "I drink because I'm bored" from women of all ages—women with babies at home, women climbing the corporate ladder, and even empty nesters. Many of us simply haven't figured out how to spend our days with anything other than a drink filling the gaps. Victoria said, "Drinking just makes those dull, boring hours go by faster."

Does drinking pass the time? Sure. Is it the best use of our spare time? Surely not.

Today's verses remind us we don't merely live for ourselves; God placed us on this planet with an intentional purpose. When we get bored, our focus becomes "How can I pass the time?" and we start living solely for ourselves. In her study guide *Get Out of Your Head: A Study in Philippians,* Jennie Allen wrote, "You and I were made to be part of an eternal story centered on the unyielding purpose of our service to an unmatched God. We were meant to live intentionally rather than floating around trying to be comfy."[1]

Our world treats boredom like it's something to run from, but it's really one of our greatest gateways to living life more fully. Boredom is your invitation to take a break, pray, read a good book, or journal and is your chance to do something good for yourself or for someone else. If you have the luxury of extra time, there are so many restorative things that you can do to fill that time. You, my friend, were meant for so much more than drinking to pass the time.

FINDING GOD'S PURPOSE

Never in a million years did I imagine myself as a sobriety coach before beginning this journey. Choosing not to drink freed up so much time and allowed me to step into my purpose. I have been given the incredible opportunity to walk alongside women through their struggles and victories and tell them there is hope. But my coaching is about so much more than just avoiding alcohol. When a client realizes she has the space, energy, and time to find true fulfillment, that's when the magic happens.

Today is the day I want you to start thinking and praying about the big picture. Here are some questions that can help guide you:

What did God put you on this earth to do?
Who are you meant to serve?
Who is already listening to you?
What have you always longed to do but haven't been able to start?
Is there a group of people, a cause, or a movement that sparks your passion?
Is there something that fills you with righteous anger that you long to help fix?
What are your natural strengths?

In the immediate months after quitting drinking, each day I woke up early to go downstairs and pray. I was desperate to figure out what He had in store for me. I knew I wanted to make an impact, but I hadn't discovered coaching opportunities yet. Then, one morning I felt Him place the idea of a podcast on my heart. I had no idea what it would be about. It wasn't until two years later that the *"But Jesus Drank Wine" & Other Stories That Kept Us Stuck* podcast was born.

God may not reveal everything to you overnight. The longer you walk the alcohol-free path and leave space for Him to speak to you, the more evident His purpose for you will become.

FEEL THE FEELS

My clients often believe they are drinking because they are bored, but in reality they are avoiding feeling hard emotions. I've learned through my coaching practice that so many of us women are programmed to avoid, shut down, or fix tricky emotions that we come across. Just yesterday, I overheard a mom in a changing room tell her toddler, "Don't cry. There's no reason to cry. It's not going to fix anything."

Whether what we feel is disappointment, frustration, anger, or sadness, alcohol can be the easy-button answer. We've been conditioned over time to fix the "feelings problem" as fast as possible. We are often led to believe that our more challenging emotions are hurdles to overcome and are encouraged to employ coping mechanisms like alcohol to blur those feelings.

Research by neuroscientist Dr. Jill Bolte Taylor has shown that merely identifying and labeling our emotions can calm our amygdala, the part of the brain responsible for processing emotions.[2]

A while back, I was coaching Janet, a mom of four in Chicago, who was grieving the loss of her mother. To navigate through her layers of grief, we undertook the following exercise together. I asked Janet to place her hands on her chest and to close her eyes. I gently suggested she take a deep breath. Following this, I guided her to voice the words, "I am sad. Of course I am feeling this way; my mother just died." We both shed tears as she repeated these words, acknowledging and affirming her sadness as a natural response to the incredible loss. This simple yet powerful exercise allowed her the space to feel that feeling rather than rush to fix it, numb it, or make it go away.

What if, instead of burying our difficult feelings in alcohol, we choose to ride the waves of our emotions?

Our Creator doesn't ask us to "get over" our emotions; instead, God urges us to hand them to Him. He can handle our pain. Remember, Jesus wept. Tears carry with them cortisol, the stress hormone.[3] When we cry, we literally shed our stress. Crying can be an innate form of relief that is so much better for us than downing a glass of ethanol.

The next time you find yourself in the throes of a complex emotion, you can try the exercise I guided Janet through. Give yourself ninety seconds to:

- Identify and name your emotion (e.g., "I feel sad.")
- Allow it to pass through you without judging it—simply observing its presence
- Hand it to Jesus and ask Him to sit with you in it

This approach will not only help you better understand your emotions but also equip you to fight the need to numb yourself or avoid the raw and the vulnerable. In feeling our feelings, we can truly understand how God is moving within us.

Our lives are meant for more than merely passing the time with alcohol; they are meant for intentional living, purposeful service, and authentic emotional experiences. By acknowledging our feelings and inviting God into our emotions, we discover a richer, more meaningful path forward—one that aligns with His divine plan and our true calling.

TiNA

ARE YOU BEGINNING TO FEEL EXCITED ABOUT WHAT God has in store for you? Take a few minutes and think on the big picture questions on page 174. Write your thoughts in your journal and then pray; tell God what you're excited about in your future and be honest about any concerns that come to mind. As you go about your day, keep your ears open to hear His response. This is only the beginning.

33

DAY THIRTY-THREE

Values Rekindled

But the Holy Spirit produces this kind of fruit in our lives: love, joy, peace, patience, kindness, goodness, faithfulness, gentleness, and self-control.

—GALATIANS 5:22–23, NLT

DURING MY SEASON OF EXCESSIVE DRINKING, I SLOWLY but surely moved further and further away from who I truly was. Drinking separated me from the values I hold dear.

I valued family, dependability, joy, faith, and honesty. But when I drank each night, none of these values were evident in my life. I wasn't reliable. I frequently chose a glass of wine over quality time with my children. I wasn't joyful, because my body was constantly being pumped with a depressant. I rarely made it to church, even though I would have told you one of my values was my faith. And I certainly wasn't being honest with myself about how my drinking was affecting my life. I compromised what was important to me because wine came first.

Ann Voskamp wrote, "When you hide who you are, you are ultimately hiding from yourself. This is a haunting, exhausting kind of lost. And if evil can keep you distracted from taking the time to ask your soul where you really are, he can take you every day further from the life you envisioned."[1]

Another value I hold dear is learning. I've always loved being a student, and I thrived in college, law school, and several other graduate programs. But during the years that my focus and energy were spent on drinking, my learning became stagnant; I was lucky if I read one book a year. But Proverbs 24:5 says, "The wise are mightier than the strong, and those with knowledge grow stronger and stronger" (NLT). With alcohol out of the way, I've thrown myself back into reading. I love finding new Bible studies, learning from mentors, and listening to podcasts that help me learn and grow.

I've mentioned before how alcohol stunted my faith. I never made it to a Sunday morning service if I had been out for cocktails the night before. Early morning wake-up calls to read the Bible and pray were nonexistent—who could be that disciplined while fighting a hangover? But now, as a sober Christian, I feel closer to Jesus than I ever have in my life. I try to prioritize my soul care, my nonnegotiable time to be with Him. I have witnessed tons of His blessings now that I am more aware and present. When I think about how God has transformed my life and that I get to share this transformation with you, I am overwhelmed with gratitude.

THE WORST KIND OF IMPOSTOR SYNDROME

One of my clients, Isla, works as a yoga instructor. During one of our remote sessions she said, "Christy, I feel like an impostor because I am teaching my yoga students all about health and wellness when I don't feel healthy myself because I'm drinking poison all the time." I wanted to reach through the screen and hug her because I could relate. If you value your health, it's hard to feel like you're living out of integrity if you're constantly drinking something that is harming your health.

When I ask my clients the question "Why do you want to take a break from alcohol?" so many of them have the same answer: "For my kids." Their children are the most important thing to them, but they feel like terrible mothers because alcohol is killing their joy, robbing them of patience, and exhausting them. Drinking can make us feel like we are living an inauthentic life because we know we're not in alignment with our values.

When I stopped drinking and started working on myself—praying a lot and asking for God's help to get me back on track—my values realigned and my connections to everyone in my life improved because I was showing up as my true, authentic self and the woman God called me to be.

Let's dive deeper into our values in today's TiNA.

TiNA

THIS IS AN IMPORTANT JOURNALING EXERCISE. PLEASE don't skip this one.

Take a minute to reflect on your values; list all the things that make you, you.

Now consider these questions:

- In what area of your life has drinking made you feel incongruent with who you truly are or want to be?
- Does drinking in any way help you stay in alignment with the values you wrote down?
- What do you need more of/less of in your life to align with your values?

Now, visualize what it might feel like to live perfectly in alignment with your values. Pray and ask God to help you refocus your life on what is truly important.

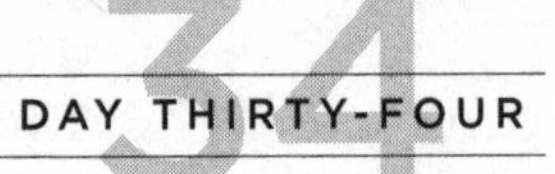

DAY THIRTY-FOUR

Meaningful Connection

The LORD himself goes before you and will be with you; he will never leave you nor forsake you. Do not be afraid; do not be discouraged.

—DEUTERONOMY 31:8

ONE OF THE REASONS I DRANK WAS BECAUSE I ASSUMED it was helping me connect with people. I drank to connect with my husband, my girlfriends, and even, in a strange way, my children because I thought that the alcohol made me a more relaxed and fun mom. If this belief resonates with you, I want you to know you're in good company. The majority of women I coach say similar things, like "I drink to socialize" or "Drinking is romantic." When I did my own alcohol fast, I had to ask myself if this story—that alcohol connected me to others—was true.

By the morning of March 9, 2020, when I cried out to Jesus for help, it was clear that alcohol had not brought me the connection I longed for. My relationships were in tatters. Chris and I were constantly bickering. I took out my grief on him, and when he didn't understand, I drank more to cope with the tension. I constantly chose to go out and party with girlfriends to numb the pain instead of being at home with Chris and the children. As a result, my family bonds were broken. My relationship with God was next to nonexistent. I had never felt so alone. I was utterly disconnected.

Alcohol's effect on connection was never more evident than in my relationship with my mom, Terry. When I was growing up, she never drank a drop of alcohol. She was my best friend. She was always included in get-togethers with my friends. Our house was the sleepover house and the house that everyone got ready for prom at. My friends would come over and knock on the door knowing she would let them in to use the pool or have a snack even if I wasn't home.

She volunteered at homeless shelters, fostered kids who needed a home, and anonymously paid tuition for a girl at my school whose parents could no longer afford it. She drove us an hour to and from church every Sunday because she wanted us to hear her favorite pastor. She was selfless, generous, and kind. When I was little, we took trips together to Disneyland and Palm Springs, and later, when I was older, to Mexico and Europe. We called our trips MDTs (Mother-Daughter Trips), and I loved them. I adored her with my whole heart.

It wasn't until I turned twenty-four that she began drinking. Her personality changed, and she shifted into a person I did not recognize. She became bitter, angry, and sad. When I got engaged, she became furious. And when I told her that Chris and I were moving to London, she told me I was abandoning her and choosing Chris over her. It broke my heart. To cope with her words, I drank. I know that my drinking further damaged our relationship because I never approached her with any compassion, grace, or forgiveness. Instead, I became angry and sad at how she had changed.

When she passed away, I mourned two people—my best friend and this mom who had hurt me deeply beyond words. Alcohol literally destroyed our relationship on both ends.

ALCOHOL FURTHER ERODED TRUE CONNECTION

It wasn't just my relationship with my mom that was affected by my alcohol. When I stopped drinking, I realized that the conversations I was having with my girlfriends over bottles of wine were the same conversation, night after night. At the time, these heavy conversations after multiple drinks seemed therapeutic, like the alcohol allowed us to express ourselves and connected us. But I realized that nothing actually felt better the next day. If anything, I felt worse. And on top of that, we never really remembered half of what we talked about. How could this be genuine, authentic connection?

One of my London-based clients, Natalie, a single, highly successful attorney, had this observation during one of our sessions: "How can my friendships be based on real connection when I am so embarrassed over my drunken behavior during a night out that I avoid seeing them for several weeks?"

I prompted, "Maybe we need to figure out what connection really means to you?" This is one of the key questions to ask ourselves along this journey.

VULNERABILITY IS KEY

I've learned that vulnerability is the cornerstone of connection. Connection is about stripping the facade that alcohol encourages us to wear and sharing our authentic selves. It's about the tender, honest exchanges that build true intimacy and trust.

I've spoken to so many clients who are worried about what their good friends will think of their sobriety, and my question back to them is, "But have you really spoken to them about how alcohol is making you feel? How it's getting in the way?" The answer is usually no. We shy away from being truly open with our journey because we struggle with vulnerability. (Shame weighs in here, too, which we will discuss on day thirty-six.)

Sobriety offers us a unique opportunity; it allows us to reevaluate our relationships, celebrate the special people in our lives, and nurture deeper connections. If you ever feel stuck or disconnected in certain relationships—with a spouse, child, parent, or friend—know that open, honest conversations and the power of prayer can heal and reconnect you with the people you hold dear. Through this journey, we can discover the true meaning of connection and strengthen the bonds that matter most.

TiNA

MAKE A LIST OF THE FIVE PEOPLE YOU'RE CLOSEST with. Write down the impact alcohol has had on each of those relationships. Consider how being more present and vulnerable might cultivate stronger connections with these people you hold most dear. If you fear that your decision to not drink or drink less will negatively affect your connection with anyone on your list, reflect on why you feel that way. End your journaling session in prayer and ask God for guidance in your relationships.

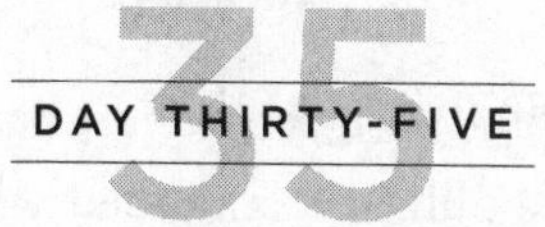

DAY THIRTY-FIVE

Alcohol and the Office

"For I know the plans I have for you," declares the LORD, *"plans to prosper you and not to harm you, plans to give you hope and a future."*

—JEREMIAH 29:11

THERE WAS AN EPISODE OF *FRIENDS* THAT YOU MIGHT REmember. In it, Rachel starts a new job and observes that her boss and colleagues frequently go outside to take cigarette breaks. To fit in and make sure she is involved in important conversations, Rachel starts smoking too. She detests the habit but feels like she has to pretend in order to gain a leg up at the office.[1]

I thought about this episode while coaching my client Erica, the CMO of a successful start-up. Erica was often at dinners with influential client executives. She texted me one morning, "I caved. I was at a wine-pairing dinner and couldn't say no because of who I was sitting with. It would have been rude and wouldn't have been good for business."

When you look at the average workplace—whether it's law, advertising, marketing, medicine, you name it—alcohol is ubiquitous. It's a recruiting tool to bring new people into the company, a marketing tactic to win new business, and a team-building method to bring colleagues together. At 6:01 P.M. in the UK, the pubs are crammed with professionals in work attire letting off steam after a long day. How we view alcohol's role in the workplace and with colleagues supports the stories we have created in our minds that we need it to fit in and achieve success.

However, in my coaching experience, I've found that women who practice sobriety enhance their performance and have a better work-life balance. Here's why.

FIVE WAYS SOBRIETY ENHANCES PERFORMANCE

Alcohol is often perceived as a key to success, but a study published in March 2022 found that alcohol results in over 232 million missed workdays every year.[2] That can't be good for business. Here are five reasons why opting out of alcohol can make you a better employee and colleague.

1. Better Decision-Making: Drinking alcohol can impair cognitive functions and decrease the ability to think critically. On the other hand, not drinking means the brain operates at its best; it's able to maintain sharp problem-solving skills and strategic decision-making. And it's not just binge drinking that can negatively affect your performance at the office; one study published in the journal *Neuropsychopharmacology* found that even moderate alcohol consumption can cause cognitive impairments that affect the brain's ability to process information.[3]

2. Improved Memory and Learning: Alcohol interferes with the hippocampus, the part of your brain responsible for memory. Abstaining from alcohol means an increase in the brain's ability to form new memories, enabling you to track more details over a more extended period of time. Drinking also may get in the way of your ability to learn, according to a comprehensive review in *Alcohol Research and Health*.[4]
3. Better Sleep: By not drinking, you can achieve deeper, more restful sleep, which enables keen alertness and stronger focus.
4. Reduced Anxiety: Alcohol affects the balance of neurotransmitters in the brain, leading to mood swings, depression, and heightened anxiety over time. Not drinking allows the brain's hormone levels to stabilize, promoting a more consistent mood and sense of well-being. This stable mental state strengthens your communication, teamwork, and leadership effectiveness.
5. Increased Energy and Stamina: Regular alcohol consumption can leave individuals feeling sluggish and fatigued. In contrast, my clients who take a substantial break from alcohol tell me how much energy they have. This energy boost may translate to better endurance in tackling work tasks, more extended periods of concentration, and more proactive solutions to those tricky problems that pop up at your desk.

YOU CAN LEAVE THE OFFICE PARTY EARLY

One of my clients, Kendall, works in sales for a large national corporation in Chicago and assumed that wine was helping her through long nights of networking. "All the small talk and sales boasting is exhausting. Numbing myself was preferable," she said. But after spending a night drowning out the small talk with multiple glasses of wine, Kendall would feel awful the next morning. "I always have a hard time getting up the next day and wonder what I'd said," she told me.

Because practice makes perfect, I tasked her with attending the next work event armed with a curiosity mindset and trying it alcohol-free. She returned to our next session with her suspicions confirmed: She just really didn't like making small talk at work events. She would rather leave early.

Kendall now continues to attend the gatherings but always has an escape plan in place. If she has to travel for a conference, she makes sure to pack things for her hotel room, like a good book, a face mask, or chocolate. Sometimes she has a great movie downloaded and ready to watch. This way, abstaining from the company drinks is even more appealing for her. She wakes up feeling great the next day and never regrets saying no to the wine.

Again, one of our most valuable tools is boundaries. And you can flex yours in a variety of ways in your professional setting.

You can leave the happy hour early. You can say no to the office wine tasting or bring along your own nonalcoholic options. You can suggest alternative activities to bond and connect with colleagues. I like to think that because of all the recent research, especially related to our health, one day we will see peer pressure to drink at the office and feel like we did when we watched Rachel in that episode of *Friends,* rooting for her not to smoke because of how it negatively affects us. But until then, we just have to concentrate on sticking to our boundaries and working together to create an environment in the workplace where everyone feels comfortable and supported, especially if we make the decision not to drink.

YOU ALWAYS HAVE A CHOICE, EVEN AT THE OFFICE

When Erica texted me that she didn't have a choice at that table full of executives, I challenged her with the question, "What else could be true here?"

I could tell that she was struggling with this question because the pressure to drink was very real for her. The root of the issue was what her colleagues were going to think of her. Erica isn't alone in this fear. Another client, Samantha, told me, "Once at a work event I was handed a beer by someone who didn't really know me, and I took a sip out of obligation because I felt like I had to."

In my own journey I realized that the sooner I could let go of the fear of what other people would think about my decision not to drink, the sooner I would find freedom from alcohol. This takes time, practice, and the continued effort of taking our thoughts captive. It *might* be true that your boss will favor your colleague who does drink, or you may miss out on signing that new client. But we need to take a look at what is *also* true.

Better decision-making, improved memory, better sleep,

reduced anxiety, and increased energy can be true for you, leading to you performing better at work, impressing your boss and colleagues, and therefore excelling in your field. It could also be true that by not drinking, you start connecting better with colleagues because you are present for the real, important conversations that matter and are home from a happy hour before the part of the night that no one remembers anyway. Be open to the truth that God already knows the plan He has for you, and that includes your career. I promise you He's not going to let your decision not to drink get in the way of the goodness He has planned for you.

TiNA

WHAT KIND OF PRESENCE DOES ALCOHOL HAVE AT your job and work culture? What challenges does not drinking pose for you? Consider what is *also* true and journal about how you can incorporate boundaries to help you navigate these challenges.

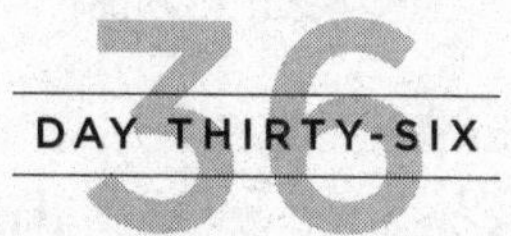

DAY THIRTY-SIX

Breaking the Chains of Shame

Therefore, there is now no condemnation [no guilty verdict, no punishment] for those who are in Christ Jesus [who believe in Him as personal Lord and Savior].

—ROMANS 8:1, AMP

ONE SPRING AFTERNOON IN LONDON, THE KIDS AND I were at a girlfriend's house for a barbecue. The moms were drinking wine in the garden, and the kids were playing happily. We carried on late into the evening. I didn't want the night to end, but I could tell my children were tired. I had the *genius* idea of everyone having a sleepover so the moms could keep drinking.

A little while later, I found Carter, six years old at the time, in the corner of a bedroom with his head in his hands, sobbing. "Mommy, I just want to go home and sleep in my own bed." I tried to convince him that it would be much more fun if he stayed. I begged him to stop crying and try to sleep—all so I could keep downing the wine.

Now, I get teary when I remember looking into his pleading big blue eyes and still choosing wine over him. I used to hold so much shame over that night and drink more to make that sting go away.

To break free from the shame cycle, it's important to remember that we live in a society that glamorizes alcohol but then shames anyone hooked on it. But here's the thing: Shame and guilt keep us stuck. Grace and compassion set us free.

SHAME HIJACKS THE BRAIN

Curt Thompson, MD, author of *The Soul of Shame,* eloquently captures the debilitating effects of shame, stating, "When I experience shame, I find it virtually impossible to turn my attention to something other than what I am feeling. I can become overwhelmed . . . and my PFC (prefrontal cortex) goes offline." He says when shame takes over, "I am unable to tell the whole story, certainly not one in which I am loved by God unconditionally and life, in the end, will be okay. My state of mind is fully disrupted, and transitioning back to one of coherence and peacefulness requires enormous effort."[1]

When we experience shame as a result of our drinking habits, it hijacks our upper-brain functions, plunging us into the survival mode of the lower brain. As we know, in this state, rational thinking becomes elusive. Our ability to see ourselves as loved and worthy is clouded.

When I was experiencing shame like this, I looked for immediate safety and solace, typically in another glass of wine. It's a common response I've also seen with numerous clients—we often try to numb the pain of shame through the temporary distraction of more alcohol. The key to breaking free from this cycle lies in challenging those shameful thoughts with the truth that we are unconditionally loved by God.

Each time we berate ourselves for drinking, we make it

much harder on ourselves to make better-informed decisions about alcohol. The encouraging news is we can break free from this cycle. Over time, and with the help of consistency, resilience, and God's love and grace, we can learn to quiet the shame.

FORGIVENESS

A few months after I stopped drinking, I started to dwell on all the mistakes I'd made—the fights with my husband that I wish I could take back and the times when I inadvertently communicated to my children that alcohol was more important than them. I asked for forgiveness and dove into the Bible, and when I did, I was reminded of Mary Magdalene in Luke 8.

You may remember this Mary as a friend of Jesus, the first human to see Him resurrected (Mark 16:9), and the woman given the most important task of all time: sharing the good news that He was alive (Mark 16:7). But it was the *way* that the Bible introduces Mary Magdalene that caught my attention:

> After this, Jesus traveled about from one town and village to another, proclaiming the good news of the kingdom of God. The Twelve were with him, and also some women who had been cured of evil spirits and diseases: Mary (called Magdalene) from whom seven demons had come out. (Luke 8:1–2)

God didn't assign the most important job in history, sharing that He rose from the dead, to a perfect woman who never struggled. God chose a woman who had seven demons cast out of her. She was a sinner, like me, who had struggled and needed God's redemption.

Jess Connolly wrote: "Maybe we need a quick shake in order to remember that when the transformative power of Jesus Christ meets painfully dark and heavy brokenness, He doesn't just *slightly* clean it up. He doesn't merely do some tidying. He doesn't sweep the grossest stuff under the rug. And He never, ever passes by brokenness in order to play with the more manageable kids on the playground."[2] Connolly reminds us that the women of the resurrection, the ones called to spread the good news that Jesus is who He says He is, were broken women, like you and me.

A NOTE ON GROWTH POINTS

If you're finding it challenging to stick to this fast and are still having growth points, then I want to encourage you to try to let go of any shame associated with the choice to drink while you're trying to improve your relationship with alcohol. After you've stepped into awareness and curiosity, each time you drink is an opportunity to learn and grow, whether during these forty days or beyond. Anytime you have a drink, ask the question: *How is this truly making me feel?*

I began to think more about God's redemption and plan for my life as He relieved me of my shame. I now realize every single experience, even the messy and shameful ones, brought me to a point where I was ready for a real change. Every drink I had taught me that alcohol was no longer serving me. I wouldn't be where I am today without the path that brought me here. God has a unique path for you too. Don't let shame hold you back from moving forward.

TiNA

TODAY, I WANT YOU TO WRITE A LETTER OF FORGIVEness to yourself. This is a chance to let go of any residual shame, guilt, and past mistakes and fully embrace the forgiveness God has given you. Here are some prompts to help guide you through this process:

1. This is a letter to yourself, for your eyes only. Start by writing your name.
2. Describe the situation(s) you're holding on to: What happened that caused you regret? Write it down as factually as you can.
3. Acknowledge how the situation(s) made you feel.
4. Recognize your mistakes. What role did you play in these situations? Again, be factual and honest.
5. Reflect on what you know now that you didn't know then.
6. Now turn your thoughts to how God has forgiven you. Maybe include Romans 8:1, our verse for the day, in your letter.
7. Next, write your own statement of forgiveness. End the letter by clearly stating, "(*Your Name*), I forgive you."
8. Take your letter to God. Pray over it. Ask the Lord to help remove your shame. Lay your forgiveness letter at His feet and be still to receive His grace.

37

DAY THIRTY-SEVEN

Sobering Up to Mommy Wine Culture

Do not love the world or anything in the world. If anyone loves the world, love for the Father is not in them.

—1 JOHN 2:15

IN LATE 2020, THE WORLD WAS VERY MUCH IN THE MIDDLE OF Covid lockdowns, and parents everywhere were stuck inside with their children, trying to homeschool while also working and ensuring everyone in the house was fed, bathed, and not spending too much time on iPads. It was at this time that Tropicana released an ad campaign showing celebrities like Molly Sims, Gabrielle Union, and Jerry O'Connell shutting themselves in a room of the house with a mini-fridge (disguised as a household item like a toolbox or laundry hamper) full of orange juice and little bottles of sparkling wine. In one ad, Molly hid in her closet, made herself a mimosa from her secret stash, and said, "It's so I can be a better mom. The best mom." The campaign used the hashtag #TakeAMimoment.

I felt shock and rage. How could a company as massive as Tropicana tell moms that they needed a mimosa to deal with their kids during a global pandemic? How would that help anything? Thankfully, I wasn't the only one enraged. The sober and sober-curious community sent strongly worded messages to Tropicana to the point where the orange juice giant apologized and took down the ads.[1]

Mommy wine culture, rampant during the pandemic, was evident in memes and posts that depicted alcohol as the only way to survive lockdown. I'll never forget one Instagram post that showed a grocery-store wine aisle with a giant sign over it that read "Homeschool Supplies."

You may not have heard the term "mommy wine culture," but you likely know what I'm talking about. Just think back to a time when you were strolling through Target. Did you happen to catch the messaging on cards, bibs, baby onesies, glassware, and Yeti tumblers that read something like:

> "I Wine Because My Kids Whine"
> "Surviving Motherhood, One Glass at a Time"
> "A mother's sacrifice isn't giving birth; it's nine months without wine."

In 2021, *Good Housekeeping* reported that there were over sixty-seven thousand "wine mom" products available for sale on Etsy,[2] even though revelations from the Centers for Disease Control and Prevention reported that the rates of excessive drinking-related deaths among women were skyrocketing.[3] Erin Stewart, MSW, a therapist who focuses on motherhood and alcohol addiction, says, "Wine mom culture says that the best and the only way to mom is with a glass of wine in hand. But it also tells us that motherhood and parenting little ones, is unbearable and brutal without the 'mommy juice' to ease the tantrums, the messes, lack of sleep, and the overwhelm of it all."[4]

Big alcohol and brands that partner with them to create these products make tons of money playing into mommy wine culture. But in addition to these efforts, women perpetuate the message through social media by sharing memes, liking the posts, and paying attention to the ads. A reel I saw on Instagram showed a mom cutting a tea bag string so that it hangs out of her Yeti, which she then fills with wine to trick everyone into thinking that she's drinking tea instead of alcohol. The text reads, "Where are all my sports moms at??" At the time of writing this, it has nearly eight million views and over one hundred thousand likes.[5] Every like of that photo is a vote that this messaging is funny and should continue to be promoted to exhausted mothers.

Another reel by a mom influencer I once came across showed her tiptoeing out of the house as her kids asked her where she was going. She told them she'd be right back, saying something along the lines of "just going out for one quick drink." But the reel made a joke of the fact that of course it wasn't just one drink because her husband had to pick her up at the bar hours later. It's supposed to be funny, hundreds of comments said so, and I would have thought it was hilarious before I stopped drinking. Now, I look at these posts much differently.

This type of content makes light of moms relying on alcohol to get through the day. But what if we switched out the substance for which the mother is sneaking out the door? What if she was sneaking out from her kids to take "just one" line of cocaine? Is it funny then? Why not? Because we have been conditioned to believe that alcohol is somehow not as addictive or as dangerous, even though it kills more people each year than cocaine and heroin combined.[6] But still, alcohol is promoted as the must-have elixir for motherhood.

THE PROBLEM

I used to think this stuff was cute. I bought the greeting cards; I gifted the tumblers. But something happened when I saw those Tropicana ads. I realized this narrative teaches us that we, as mothers, need to medicate ourselves to deal with our kids because they're tough work, they're too hard to handle. And our children see this narrative in our behavior. They understand more than we think. My client Michelle said, "It broke my heart to think my daughter would believe she was the reason I drank."

If you aren't a mother, this topic is still super important. It affects your mother, sisters, nieces and nephews, godchildren, cousins, and friends. It's not just a message to mothers; it's a message to children.

When I was drinking, I was fuzzy through so many special moments. I wish I could have been fully present. As the saying goes: The days are long, but the years are short. And I missed so much.

My children, starting when they were four, have attended a beach summer camp each year in Santa Monica. They are put in groups with a different color shirt depending on their age group. I remember going to drop off the kids the year I quit drinking and looking out at all the different colored shirts—from toddlers to preteens. My eyes welled up with tears as I realized I had missed many of those years because I chose to sit on my sun lounger and drink rosé. Sure, I was there, but I wasn't *really*.

I think about how hard I prayed for my two children before they were even born, how I asked the Lord for them to be healthy, and He blessed me with them. And it makes me sad to think about the times I promoted the message that they were a burden.

Please don't get me wrong. Being a mom is hard. It's the most demanding job ever. I thought the baby years were tough, but nothing prepared me for the tween and teen years, and I'm only at the beginning.

But there are other ways to find rest from and reward for motherhood that don't involve wine. First, make sure you are taking care of yourself. This can be difficult if your kids are tiny, but even simple shifts like going to bed early, asking for help from family members, and doing activities you really love with your kids can make a big difference.

As the apostle Paul reminds us in Philippians 4:13, "I can do all things through him who strengthens me" (ESV). With God's help, we not only can endure motherhood's challenging seasons but thrive in them. We don't need to medicate ourselves with alcohol; instead, we can seek solace, rest, and reward in healthier ways. It's okay if those ways don't seem immediately apparent to you right now. I encourage you today to stay in experiment mode, and you'll uncover ways to cope.

By focusing our attention on God and relying on His strength, we can rise above the harmful narratives and provide our children with the very best gift—being fully present with them as they grow up.

TiNA

IF YOU'RE ON SOCIAL MEDIA AND SEE A MEME OR A VIDEO making light of mommy wine culture, don't share it. Feel free to unfollow accounts that glamorize drinking as a coping mechanism for parenting. Begin to step into awareness about this messaging and ask our core question, "Is this true?" Next time you're in your local Target or on Etsy, take notice of the items that tie in alcohol to parenting. Meditate on Romans 12:2, which says, "Don't become so well-adjusted to your culture that you fit into it without even thinking. Instead, fix your attention on God. You'll be changed from the inside out. . . . Unlike the culture around you, always dragging you down . . . God brings the best out of you" (MSG).

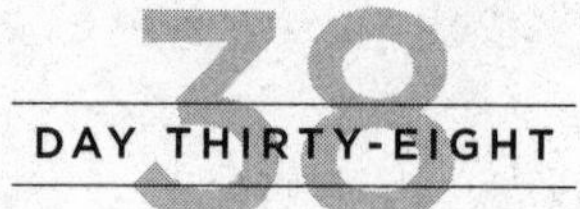

DAY THIRTY-EIGHT

Travel and Vacations Without Alcohol

He said to them, "Come with me by yourselves to a quiet place and get some rest."

—MARK 6:31

As an American expat living in London, I've spent a lot of time on airplanes, especially when the kids were tiny and not stuck to a school schedule, flying back and forth between London and Los Angeles. I always drank wine throughout the flight to "calm" my nerves about having little children on a long flight. I would arrive in Los Angeles after a very long day on a plane and be completely jet-lagged, partially hungover, or maybe even still a little buzzed.

Then came my first sober long-haul flight. Granted, the kids were older, so it wasn't as tricky, but I remember standing at baggage claim at LAX and not feeling like I wanted to crawl into a hole and die. Instead, I had some semblance of energy. Going without alcohol made the jet lag so much easier. It gave me more patience with the children. The difference was incredible. Travel was already hard enough, especially with two children in tow, and I realized that I had made it harder on myself when I drank wine throughout the flight.

THE AIRPORT AND THE AIRPLANE

I worked with a client, Kathryn, in New York City. She was a high-ranking executive who traveled all the time for work. Initially, the Achilles' heel of her alcohol fast was the airport lounge and the airplane. She usually traveled business class and struggled to disassociate wine from the pressure of traveling. She longed for a treat or reward for working so hard, so we slowly started working on substitutes for drinking on the airplane. Putting away her laptop and allowing herself to switch off and watch a movie or read a book was a great substitute because it meant her mind was getting a break from work. She also started bringing her favorite snacks on her flights so she could have something to munch on that felt like a treat but wouldn't cause her to reach her destination feeling totally zonked.

The airport lounge is another place where she struggled, and boy, could I relate. I would often start my trips to the US or anywhere else with a glass of champagne in the lounge. However, nobody tells you that a glass of champagne will make you want to drink throughout the entire day of travel. When Kathryn realized that drinking at the airport would start her off on the wrong foot for her trip, she was ready to pass on the preflight cocktail.

If you're a nervous traveler, remember that alcohol spikes our adrenaline and cortisol, making the whole experience more stressful, not less. Flying already dehydrates us due to the air pressure in the cabin, so when we drink, we are doubly dehydrating ourselves. The wine also contributes to jet lag (or exhaustion) because our bodies may absorb less oxygen when we drink, which causes us to feel more fatigued. And then there's the havoc that flying wreaks on your digestion because of cabin pressure changes.[1] Add alcohol to the mix, and you're creating a recipe for an upset stomach.

IT GETS EASIER

I've coached many women through their first alcohol-free vacation. It's a big milestone, and once you've got one alcohol-free vacation under your belt, you'll find it gets a lot easier. One summer, Chris and I surprised the kids with a Disney cruise through some amazing Nordic countries. The boat's pickup spot was Copenhagen. I'd never been there and was so excited to see the city and surprise the children by stumbling across the "Mickey boat" in the harbor.

I was frantically packing the night before we left. So how did I ease my travel tensions? You guessed it; I poured myself a glass of wine. I don't know how many I had, but it was enough to have a disrupted sleep. I woke up on the day we were leaving and felt exhausted. By the time we got to Copenhagen, I was wrecked. I asked Chris if he could take the children to dinner so I could rest. There's a photo of Ella and Carter in a park with ice cream. The lighting is perfect, and it's one of my favorite photos. But I wasn't there because I was too tired. I never saw Copenhagen; we got on the ship the next day. There are other European cities I have not properly seen because the vacation involved so much drinking that I skipped shows, museums, and must-see moments to keep drinking wine or sleep it off.

We are deeply conditioned to believe alcohol is essential to a vacation. How often have you uttered the phrase "I need a vacation from my vacation" because you come home exhausted? I've done that so many times. We go on vacation to rest, to get a break, but then we end up sabotaging our rest. We schedule a getaway to connect with our family, but the alcohol makes us disconnected.

DON'T FORGET YOUR BOUNDARIES

I received a photo from my client Amanda while she was on vacation in Mexico with her family. It was a picture of the adult pool. Alcohol was everywhere, just as you would expect it to be at a hotel in Mexico during spring break. "Too much alcohol. I'm relocating," she wrote. She later sent me a photo of the quiet pool at the same resort. "This I can do," she said. When it comes to vacations, you may need to mindfully make choices, like where your sun lounger is located, to give yourself the opportunity to rest.

Another client, Elsa, had booked a trip to South African wine country before we started working together. She was panicking about going on the trip but didn't want to cancel. We tweaked her itinerary and substituted massages and walking trails for some of the wine-tasting times. After she returned from her trip, she told me she was thrilled that just by making these few minor, well-thought-out adjustments ahead of time, she was able to go on her trip, have a great time with her friends, and not feel pressured to drink the entire time.

EXPECTATIONS

My first proper vacation (or "holiday" as they say here in the UK) was to Zakynthos, Greece. By this point, I was six months alcohol-free, and Jesus and I had done a ton of work on my mindset. I had prayed about it and decided I wouldn't be apprehensive about this vacation. I set my expectations ahead of time that this was going to be fun, even if it was different. I chose to be excited about my first alcohol-free vacation with my children in Europe. I looked forward to sunshine, a kids' club, and lots of feta and tzatziki. I wasn't going to let the absence of rosé ruin all of that for me.

We checked in to our hotel and settled in for the week. That first sober holiday was magical. Watching the children laugh, play, and jump in the ocean made my heart feel incredibly full. Enjoying the delicious Greek food without numbing my taste buds with wine felt like an entirely new experience. Lying in the sun and feeling the warmth without a wine buzz was incredible. Being positive and setting those expectations before the trip meant I could experience all the blessings of a vacation without worrying about alcohol. If you go into an alcohol-free first, vacation or otherwise, expecting it to be awful, it probably will be awful. Remember to focus not on what you're giving up but on what you're gaining.

WHAT MAKES A VACATION A VACATION?

Let's redefine what makes a vacation a vacation. It's not about alcohol; it's about enjoying the beauty of God's creation, savoring delicious cuisine, cherishing the precious time spent with loved ones, and getting much-needed rest. By embracing travel without booze, these things are possible. By skipping the alcohol, you open the door to a world of enriching experiences where every sunset, every laughter-filled day, and every genuine connection become lasting memories.

TiNA

When was the last time you said or felt you needed a "vacation from your vacation"? As you think back, ask yourself, did alcohol enhance or detract from your trip? Journal your fears about letting go of alcohol on vacation. Ask yourself, "What am I assuming about a vacation without alcohol?"

If you have a trip coming up, ask, "How do I want to feel at the end of this vacation?" And then determine if alcohol can genuinely support you in how you want to feel.

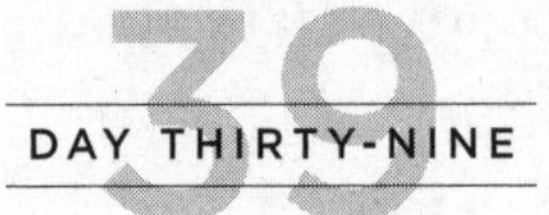

DAY THIRTY-NINE

Fixated or Free?

> *Now all glory to God, who is able, through his mighty power at work within us, to accomplish infinitely more than we might ask or think.*
>
> —EPHESIANS 3:20, NLT

WHILE COMPLETING ONE OF MY SOBRIETY-FOCUSED coaching certification programs, I met a woman named Sandra. We became friends through our training, but soon after I began coaching, I heard from her and learned that she had decided not to complete the course and had gone back to drinking. When we first became friends, she hadn't had a drink in eight months, but she later decided she didn't want to say no to alcohol forever; she thought she could moderate.

Sandra wound up coming to me for coaching about a year later. She'd had enough. "I thought I could keep alcohol small, but it kept getting bigger. I thought I could control it, but I can't." This incredibly strong woman had at one point fallen so in love with sobriety that she began training to coach others wanting to walk the same path. She had spent tens of thousands of dollars on training but was lured back in by the story that moderation is the key to a healthy relationship with alcohol. She believed that alcohol still held a benefit to her and that she could outsmart it, even though it is highly addictive.

Maybe you picked up this book because you just wanted to take a break from alcohol; lasting sobriety was never the goal. That's cool. I coach women all the time who come to me with the goal of moderation. For so many of them, when they learn how tricky moderation is, combined with how good they begin to feel without alcohol in their system, they realize that they would prefer to be 100 percent alcohol-free. You have choices. I would encourage you to pray about your decision to drink in moderation versus going alcohol-free. At the same time, consider the following question: Do you want to be free from alcohol, or do you want to be fixated on alcohol? Here's what I mean.

THE RULES WE CAN'T KEEP

When moderating, we constantly make (and break) rules we set for ourselves, like "I'll only have one glass," "I'll have water in between drinks," "I'll only drink on weekends," and "I won't drink alone." The problem, as you now know, is that it's impossible to stick to those rules because of the addictive nature of alcohol. We try to drink less but end up fixated on alcohol. We're constantly attempting to manage our alcohol intake, and as a result, alcohol becomes our focus. Alcohol is in the driver's seat.

One of my attempts at moderation looked like this: When trying to drink less and save calories, I switched from drinking red wine at night to making my ranch water at home:

tequila with sparkling water and lime. I thought this was much better than three or four glasses of wine because initially, I could only physically have one or two tequilas. The problem was that one or two tequilas quickly turned into three, and when friends came over, it became even more. So, my goal of consuming less alcohol ended with the result of drinking even more. I raised my tolerance so much that I had to drink more and more to get that initial buzz, and I would spend the remainder of the evening chasing it. We all know how that ends.

When I stopped drinking, I realized how much mental real estate was being taken up by alcohol. I didn't want to be fixated anymore; I wanted to be liberated; I wanted to be free.

After a period of living life alcohol-free, my client Lydia made the decision to experiment with moderation on an upcoming vacation. During a call before she was set to leave for her trip, she said that even though she had decided to try moderation and we had talked it through, she wasn't sure of her choice. "I know too much now," she stated. "And even though I had already chosen to moderate, I can't stop thinking about how alcohol is going to affect my trip. I think it's better if I take alcohol off the table completely so I can have all the headspace back." The second Lydia chose to try the trip alcohol-free, her mind was free and clear to enjoy her time away, as opposed to spending all her time thinking about how the moderation game was going to play out.

Moderation often takes up way too much of our precious brain power. The only way I've found to be truly free from alcohol is not to drink it. If the option is there, alcohol will run the show in your mind.

THE MODERATION UNICORNS DON'T HAVE TO TRY TO MODERATE

I have a friend, Suzie, who would always come to a dinner or night out, have one drink, and leave it at that. On a "wild night," she would have two. She is kind, engaging, intelligent, and so much fun to be around. She seems to have the moderation thing perfected. During my first year of sobriety, I couldn't stop wondering about how she did it.

It must be me, I thought. *I must just be doing this wrong. I just need to stick to the two glasses. Two glasses must be the answer.* I got wrapped up in comparing myself with other friends, watching them moderate and wondering why I couldn't do it.

It's important to talk about comparison when it comes to this journey. You've heard the expression that comparison is the thief of joy, and it also applies to our drinking journeys. Just because everyone else drinks doesn't mean it's good for us.

Comparison is modern-day coveting. One of the Ten Commandments is not coveting or desiring what someone else has (Exodus 20:17). And boy, was I coveting other people's ability to drink in moderation! I wasn't supposed to be comparing my drinking to Suzie's; I was meant to figure out if alcohol was getting in the way of the life God had called me to. So often, we get tripped up by other people and what they are doing. It might seem like everyone around you can moderate, but the reality is that each person has a totally different relationship with alcohol.

Remember, these moderation unicorns never saw the benefit in alcohol the same way as you and I have, so the pull for them to drink isn't the same. They don't use alcohol to cope, unwind, or relax to the extent we do. Maybe they use one glass to celebrate or relax, but it stops at one. Moderation unicorns don't have to try to moderate. They have not given alcohol a job in the same way.

The other significant thing to remember about people who can seemingly moderate is that we have no idea what's going on in their heads. My friend Suzie could take or leave the cocktails because she was not relying on the effects of alcohol. But there are also women out there who *look* like they can moderate, but behind the scenes, internally, their wheels are spinning. Maybe your friend is doing everything she can to stick to two drinks, and her mind is fixated on drinking rules. Just because someone may have the moderation game perfected on the outside does not mean they are *free* from alcohol if they are thinking about how to control it all the time.

Don't compare yourself to other women—the school mom, your best friend, your cousin, the woman on social media. Their paths are uniquely their own, just as yours is your own. It's easy to get caught up in wondering how they seem to have mastered moderation or seem to effortlessly enjoy a drink without it becoming an obsession. But remember, appearances can be deceiving. What matters most is the purpose-filled life God has planned for you, not how well you measure up to others.

As our fast is coming to an end, know that you have the power, with the help of the Holy Spirit, to break free from the fixation on alcohol. You can reclaim the mental real estate it once occupied and use it for the things that truly matter. As our verse today says, we are capable of immeasurably more than we can imagine, *according to His power.* Keep moving forward with faith, and you'll find the strength to leave your fixation on alcohol behind and embrace the freedom He has for you.

TiNA

TAKE SOME TIME TODAY AND MEDITATE ON THIS question: "Do I want to be fixated on alcohol or free from alcohol?"

The following exercise can be really helpful in showing you how much time and space alcohol has taken up for you. The goal here is to determine the percentage of your time spent on booze.

You've got 168 hours in one week. First, figure out how many hours you're awake. If you sleep eight hours each night, subtract fifty-six hours:

168 (TOTAL HOURS) – 56 (SLEEPING HOURS) = 112

Now estimate how many hours are spent drinking, thinking about drinking, buying alcohol, and recovering from hangovers.

When I did this exercise a few years back, I calculated I spent about five to six hours each day either drinking, thinking about drinking, or recovering from drinking.

Take however many hours you spend per week drinking and thinking about drinking, divide it by your waking hours, and multiply by 100 to get the percentage of waking hours spent on alcohol:

35 (HOURS SPENT ON DRINKING)
÷ 112 (WAKING HOURS) = 0.31.
Then you multiply by 100,
and you get 31 percent.

I was spending over 31 percent of my *life* on alcohol.

As you think about how you want to move forward after this forty-day fast, remember this number and consider how best you want to spend this percentage of the life God has given you.

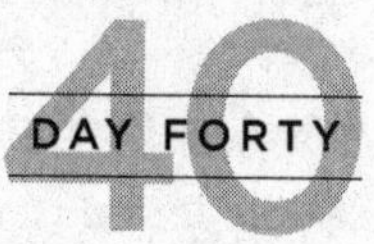

Reflections on the Journey

In all my prayers for all of you, I always pray with joy because of your partnership in the gospel from the first day until now, being confident of this, that he who began a good work in you will carry it on to completion until the day of Christ Jesus.

—PHILIPPIANS 1:4–6

CONGRATULATIONS ON COMING TO THE END OF YOUR forty-day alcohol fast! Whether you went all forty days without drinking or you had a few growth points along the way, I hope you spend time today honoring and celebrating the work you've done. This is just the beginning. You can't unknow what you know now. Since you've uncovered the real reasons why you were drinking and learned how alcohol truly affects you and how it may be getting in the way of designing a life you love, you get to decide, with God's help, how you want alcohol to show up for you going forward.

HOW MUCH DID YOU SAVE?

Go back and count the number of days that you remained alcohol-free and celebrate those days. Be proud!

Then, calculate how much money you saved by not drinking. Multiply the number of dollars you'd normally spend on a bottle of wine or cocktails in a day by the number of days you've stayed alcohol-free and total it up. For example, if you haven't had anything to drink for thirty-six of the last forty days and would typically spend fifteen dollars a day on a bottle of wine, you've saved $540.

At the time of writing this chapter, I have not had anything to drink for 1,240 days. I used to spend around twenty dollars a day on alcohol, so I've saved $24,800.

Now go back and total the number of hours saved. If you're anything like me, drinking took up a lot of time. I had to factor in not only the hours that I was drinking but also the hours lost to hangovers. Take the number of days you've stayed alcohol-free and multiply it by the number of hours a day you previously would have spent on alcohol. Those hours can eventually total up to weeks, months, even years. At the time of writing, I have saved seven months of my life. I am so grateful I can now be so intentional with my time and money. *Thank You, Jesus.*

IT'S ABOUT SO MUCH MORE THAN ALCOHOL

I was chatting with my client Scarlett about her list of reasons why she likes to drink. Like so many ladies I speak with, she had used alcohol to cope with a challenging situation in her life. As she told me her story, she stopped midsentence, and tears formed in her eyes. "Oh, wow," she said. "It's not actually about the wine, is it?"

I smiled and shook my head. "Nope. It's got nothing to do with wine."

See, here's the thing. The alcohol isn't the point. It's not about how many glasses of that wine you drink, when you drink them, or how often you drink them. It's about why you're drinking. The reasons vary from person to person. Whatever your reasons are, now that you've completed this part of your journey, you're more aware of the "why" driving your drinking. You have stepped into awareness. And on the other side of awareness is where freedom lives. When we get curious and ask questions, we figure out if there are better ways to handle stress, anxiety, and grief. We are able to learn better. That, my friend, is what this whole thing is about—about getting to know yourself and growing into the woman God wants you to be.

I want you to return to your list of reasons why you assumed you like to drink that you wrote down on day six. (Seriously, don't skip this step.) Looking back at your list now, which of these beliefs have shifted and which still feel like they hold a bit of truth? For example, by week three without alcohol, I no longer believed I needed red wine to fall asleep. My sleep had improved so drastically that I would never drink for sleep again. It was the belief that I needed alcohol to have fun that took me a lot longer to turn on its head. I had to live my life without alcohol, doing all the things that I would typically do for fun. And I had to find new ways to have fun without the ethanol. Since ditching alcohol, I have danced on tables, gone on vacations, sung karaoke, had lots of date nights, and so much more. I went to Taylor Swift's The Eras Tour with Ella. It was nearly four hours of nonstop singing and dancing; we didn't get home until two in the morning. It was one of the most fun nights of my life, and alcohol didn't even cross my mind.

Each alcohol-free milestone always feels a little awkward

at first. The first barbecue, the first girls' night out, the first time hosting a baby shower, the first flight, the first vacation, the first concert, the first Christmas and birthday. At each event, I felt like a fish out of water for the first twenty minutes or so. But as weeks and months passed, those awkward minutes shortened, and I became more and more confident. Each first taught me something about myself, my loved ones, and the world around me.

Give yourself grace for this process. I don't expect you to have dismantled every single story you have about alcohol in forty days. It takes time to undo the subconscious conditioning built up over the years. The good news is it won't take you forever. Just keep at it.

WHAT DO DRINKING AND GIVING BIRTH HAVE IN COMMON?

I mentioned earlier how I used to think fondly about that one perfect beach day with my family and friends drinking rosé. A few times in my first year of sobriety, I wondered if maybe wine could have a place in my life again for days just like that one. Perhaps I could win the moderation battle and have a glass or two every once in a while. This thinking pattern is known as fading affect bias (FAB),[1] and I have seen many clients experience it over the years. Our tendency is to get a little alcohol-free time under our belt, then look back on our drinking and only remember the good, happy times. We give alcohol the credit for those good times, and we forget the sleepless nights and the hangovers. It's like when you have a baby and can only remember being handed the perfect newborn and forget the pain and discomfort of childbirth.

In reality, that perfect sunny beach day was followed by a chaotic night with the kids and a raging hangover. That beautiful day ruined my next day, but FAB made it so I only recalled the first hour or so of that memorable day.

If a few more weeks pass and you start feeling nostalgic about your drinking, I want you to remember the FAB. Instead of looking back and giving alcohol all the credit for the good times, remember to consider the whole picture. We cannot get the brief, temporary euphoria without everything that comes after.

FIND COMMUNITY

If you decide to keep your alcohol-free journey going, it is *so* important that you find community. The great news is that there are so many options for you. I coach groups of women, and there are many other great coaches and communities for you to join. Whether it's a traditional AA meeting, an online recovery community, or a group of grounded friends, make sure to find a space with people you feel safe enough to open up to. Don't be discouraged if the first or even second group or coach doesn't work. Keep trying. You will find your tribe. I promise there are incredible Christian women who can help support you with grace and compassion. I'd love to help get you connected with others. See the resources section at the end of the book for more details.

. . .

Right now, I am writing this last chapter in the same hotel room I stayed in for a week after my mother died. I am looking out at the same view—a golf course with the mountains behind it and downtown Los Angeles in full view. It's next door to where my dad lives, hence why I've landed in the exact same hotel room again while visiting him.

I remember how lost, broken, confused, and alone I felt in the days that I was waking up early in this bed in 2018. I remember one morning in particular: I looked at the five o'clock neon pink sky and the mist covering the palm trees and shook off the hangover. I opened my mom's Bible, which I had taken from her nightstand, and found Jeremiah 29:11: "'For I know the plans I have for you,' declares the Lord, 'plans to prosper you and not to harm you, plans to give you hope and a future.'"

I had no idea then what God's plans for me might be. Sitting in this same room, reading the same verse six years later, I am in total awe of what I am doing and where I am at this moment. The fact that I have been given the opportunity to write this book is moving me to tears as I type. I am no longer heartbroken and lost; I am strong. I am no longer alone; I am fully connected with my Savior. I have been blessed with meeting and coaching women all over the globe. I have virtually held their hands as they have explored a life without alcohol and, with my Christian clients, a life closer to God.

I reread that passage in Jeremiah and noticed verse 13, which says, "You will seek me and find me when you seek me with all your heart."

As we close our forty days together, that is what I most desire to leave with you: Keep seeking Him. If you do that, He will accomplish things in your life that you never could have imagined. God showed me some of His plans for me through sobriety. Maybe He has the same plan for you. But above all, I just urge you, my sweet friend, to continue to seek Him with all your heart. Because you never know what He has in store for you.

TiNA

YOU'VE COURAGEOUSLY NAVIGATED THIS FORTY-DAY journey. Each step, each growth point, has added to your strength, knowledge, and self-awareness. Even if you drank less than you normally would while reading this book, that is a *huge* win, and you should be really proud of yourself.

Today, your TiNA is twofold. First, celebrate! Do something today that marks the end of an incredible forty days of self-exploration and getting closer to Jesus. Sit down at the dinner table and share what you've accomplished with your family, or phone a friend and tell her what you've learned. I love a good old-fashioned kitchen dance party, so pop on some tunes and get to rejoicing!

Second, don't forget to snap a selfie and compare it to your day-one photo. Marvel at how your eyes may be clearer. Does your skin look more glowy? What differences do you see?

Finally, today, and all the days, seek Him. Seek Him with all your heart, whether it's continuing on into a life of sobriety after today or not. Seek Him, and He will guide you. His plans for you are good.

Resources

To receive a free personalized celebration tracker, go to lovelifesober 40dayfast.com.

For more information on one-on-one or group coaching with Christy, head to lovelifesober.co.uk/coaching.

To do the forty-day fast with friends, head to lovelifesober40dayfast.com.

To get in touch with Christy directly, email Christy@lovelifesober.co.uk or follow Christy on Instagram @lovelifesoberwithchristy.

You can listen to the *"But Jesus Drank Wine" & Other Stories That Kept Us Stuck* podcast on Apple, Spotify, and YouTube, or visit ButJesusDrank Wine.com.

Acknowledgments

CHRIS, THIS JOURNEY HAS MADE ME FALL IN LOVE WITH you all over again, as ditching alcohol allowed me to realign my values with what is most important to me: our family. Thank you for creating a safe space for me to learn more about my relationship with alcohol and cheering me on every single step of the way. Thank you for proofreading every single Instagram post I've ever written and hanging with the kids so I could write this book and build my coaching practice. I appreciate every meal you have prepared for our family and every mocktail you've ever made me. I love you beyond words.

Ella, my dear, sweet, wonderful girl. Thank you for helping me come up with the title of my practice and this book. I will never forget the day we were sitting on the couch together and you drew the heart and wrote those words, *Love, Life, Sober.* "That's it!" we said. You are the most brilliant girl I have ever met, and I love you beyond words. God gave me the best daughter when He gave me you. Happiness is blasting Taylor Swift with you all day every day.

Carter, I don't know how you got so kind. (That's not true. You got it from your dad.) You are the most wonderful son, and I am so blessed by you. Thank you for asking, "How did you sleep, Mommy?" every single morning and "How's the booking coming?" every time you see me furiously typing away. Your loving and caring heart reminds me of Jesus, and I have never known a sweeter soul.

Mom, I miss you. Every. Single. Day. Thank you for introducing me to Jesus. I am so glad I get to see you again one day.

Dad, thank you for how you love me and my family. We are so grateful for everything you do for us.

Mary DeMuth, sitting around a campfire in Switzerland hearing you pray changed my life. Thank you for taking a chance on a first-time writer and on a topic that many didn't want to touch with a ten-foot pole. I am beyond blessed by you and so honored to call you my agent and friend.

Holly, I always wanted a sister and only had to wait until I turned fifteen to get one. Your unwavering support since, well, forever, means the world to me. Thank you for everything. I'm so glad we never have to make ourselves sick from tequila ever again.

Barty, Alice, and Erin—my London babes. Because of you gals I was able to navigate all those tricky alcohol-free firsts with zero judgment. I am forever grateful to you.

Caitlin, thank you so much for your incredible support and for teaching me so much about trusting Jesus.

Katie, my dear, sweet cousin (but more like a sister), thank you for your late-night prayers from the moment I said, "I think I'm not going to drink anymore." Your words of encouragement have given me so much strength. I love you and your sweet girls so much.

Estee Zandee, thank you for allowing me to tell my story and helping me grow into a better writer. Your wisdom and advice have been invaluable to me.

Meade Holland Shirley, having a Christian sister in the coaching world has been a game changer for me. Thank you for all you have taught and continue to teach me. You have the most beautiful heart, and our podcast ministry has been a blessing I never thought possible.

Wendy McCallum, my mentor and business-building guru, thank you so much for all your wisdom, friendship, cheerleading, and so much more. You have been a massive blessing to me.

Lauren, one of my OG clients and now precious friend, I hope there will be more partner Pilates in the Cotswolds in the future. I love you, babe.

Sam, thank you for being here since the beginning and for everything you have done to support me; I hope you know how much I appreciate you.

Notes

DAY ONE: STARTING WITH GRACE

1. Amy N. Dalton and Stephen A. Spiller, "Too Much of a Good Thing: The Benefits of Implementation Intentions Depend on the Number of Goals," abstract, *Journal of Consumer Research* 39, no. 3 (October 1, 2012): 600–614, https://academic.oup.com/jcr/article-abstract/39/3/600/1822636.

DAY TWO: YOU'RE NOT ALONE

1. Thomas Pellechia, "Low- and No-Alcohol Beverages Are a Growing Trend Worldwide, Says New Report," *Forbes,* February 20, 2019, www.forbes.com/sites/thomaspellechia/2019/02/20/lowno-alcohol-beverages-are-in-the-worldwide-future-says-latest-report/?sh=75935c871c85.
2. "Is Generation Z Drinking Less?," Cleveland Clinic, October 31, 2023, https://health.clevelandclinic.org/why-gen-z-is-drinking-less.
3. Tamar Adler, "Has Everyone Stopped Drinking?," *British Vogue,* August 21, 2022, www.vogue.co.uk/arts-and-lifestyle/article/sober-curious-movement.
4. "No- and Low-Alcohol Category Value Surpasses $11bn in 2022," IWSR, www.theiwsr.com/no-and-low-alcohol-category-value-surpasses-11bn-in-2022.
5. Sabrina Weiss and Sam Burros, "Buzz-worthy Brands Without the Booze! See Which Celebrities Have Launched Non-Alcoholic Drink Lines," *People,* updated December 7, 2022, https://people.com/food/celebrity-non-alcoholic-drink-brands.

DAY FOUR: RENEWING YOUR MIND

1. Zenith Media, "Alcohol Adspend to Beat Market with 5.3% Growth in 2021 as Hospitality Opens Up," Zenith Media, May 24, 2021, www.zenithmedia.com/alcohol-adspend-to-beat-market-with-5-3-growth-in-2021-as-hospitality-opens-up.

DAY FIVE: CRACKING THE CODE

1. Anushree N. Karkhanis and Ream Al-Hasani, "Dynorphin and Its Role in Alcohol Use Disorder," *Brain Research* 1735 (March 2020): 146742, https://doi.org/10.1016/j.brainres.2020.146742.
2. Karkhanis and Al-Hasani, "Dynorphin."
3. Luke D. Vella and David Cameron-Smith, "Alcohol, Athletic Performance and Recovery," *Nutrients* 2, no. 8 (2010): 781–89, https://doi.org/10.3390/nu2080781.
4. Daniel G. Amen, *Change Your Brain, Change Your Life: The Breakthrough Program for Conquering Anxiety, Depression, Obsessiveness, Anger, and Impulsiveness* (New York: Harmony Books, 1998), 3–5.
5. Amen, *Change Your Brain,* 95–96.
6. Psalm 139:13–14.

DAY SIX: THE BATTLE IN OUR BRAINS

1. James Clear, *Atomic Habits: An Easy & Proven Way to Build Good Habits & Break Bad Ones* (New York: Avery, 2018), 48.

DAY EIGHT: TAKE EVERY THOUGHT CAPTIVE

1. Christopher Cook, *Healing What You Can't Erase: Transform Your Mental, Emotional, and Spiritual Health from the Inside Out* (New York: WaterBrook, 2024), 60.

DAY NINE: DITCHING THE LABEL

1. Raymond Walters et al., "Transancestral GWAS of Alcohol Dependence Reveals Common Genetic Underpinnings with Psychiatric Disorders," *Nature Neuroscience* 21 (November 26, 2018): 1656–69, https://doi.org/10.1038/s41593-018-0275-1.

2. "Genetics of Alcohol Use Disorder," National Institute on Alcohol Abuse and Alcoholism, accessed April 8, 2024, www.niaaa.nih.gov/alcohols-effects-health/alcohol-use-disorder/genetics-alcohol-use-disorder.

DAY ELEVEN: PRIME WITH PRAYER

1. Maverick City Music, "Promises," track 5 on *Maverick City Vol. 3 Part 1,* April 17, 2020.
2. Mark Batterson, *The Circle Maker: Praying Circles Around Your Biggest Dreams and Greatest Fears* (Grand Rapids, Mich.: Zondervan, 2011), 156.
3. Batterson, *The Circle Maker,* 156.

DAY TWELVE: UNDERSTANDING TRIGGERS AND HABITS

1. American Psychological Association, *APA Dictionary of Psychology,* s.v. "trigger," accessed April 19, 2018, https://dictionary.apa.org/trigger.
2. Amanda E. White, *Not Drinking Tonight: A Guide to Creating a Sober Life You Love* (New York: Hachette, 2022), 217–18.

DAY THIRTEEN: OVERCOME THE URGE TO DRINK

1. "HALT: Pay Attention to These Four Stressors on Your Recovery," Cleveland Clinic, May 23, 2022, https://health.clevelandclinic.org/halt-hungry-angry-lonely-tired.
2. Clare Pooley, *The Sober Diaries: How One Woman Stopped Drinking and Started Living* (London: Coronet, 2017).
3. Philippians 4:13.

DAY FOURTEEN: NAVIGATING SUGAR CRAVINGS

1. Amy N. Dalton and Stephen A. Spiller, "Too Much of a Good Thing: The Benefits of Implementation Intentions Depend on the Number of Goals," *Journal of Consumer Research* 39, no. 3 (October 1, 2012): 600–614.
2. Brooke Scheller, *How to Eat to Change How You Drink* (New York: Balance, 2023), 66.
3. Jess Connolly, *Breaking Free from Body Shame: Dare to Reclaim What God Has Named Good* (Grand Rapids, Mich.: Zondervan, 2021), 96.

DAY FIFTEEN: EMBRACING CHOICE

1. "The Cycle of Alcohol Addiction," National Institute on Alcohol Abuse and Alcoholism, 2021, www.niaaa.nih.gov/publications/cycle-alcohol-addiction.
2. For more on these models, see Marc Gelkopf, Shabtai Levitt, and Avi Bleich, "An Integration of Three Approaches to Addiction and Methadone Maintenance Treatment: The Self-Medication Hypothesis, the Disease Model and Social Criticism," *Israel Journal of Psychiatry and Related Sciences* 39, no 2 (2002): 140–51, https://pubmed.ncbi.nlm.nih.gov/12227229; "Understanding the Models of Addiction," Sequoia Behavioral Health, accessed April 13, 2024, www.sequoiabehavioralhealth.org/blogs/understanding-the-models-of-addiction.
3. Mayo Clinic Staff, "Depression in Women: Understanding the Gender Gap," Mayo Clinic, January 29, 2019, www.mayoclinic.org/diseases-conditions/depression/in-depth/depression/art-20047725.
4. "Facts & Statistics: Anxiety Disorders in Women," Anxiety and Depression Association of America, https://adaa.org/living-with-anxiety/women/facts.
5. Amy Keller, "Alcohol and Dopamine," DrugRehab.com, updated March 20, 2023, www.drugrehab.com/addiction/alcohol/alcoholism/alcohol-and-dopamine.

DAY SIXTEEN: THE ILLUSION OF SLEEP

1. Matthew Walker, *Why We Sleep: Unlocking the Power of Sleep and Dreams* (New York: Scribner, 2017), 163.
2. William Porter, *Alcohol Explained: Understand Why You Drink and How to Stop* (self-pub., CreateSpace, 2015), 44.
3. Walker, *Why We Sleep*, 269.
4. Andrew Huberman, "What Alcohol Does to Your Body, Brain & Health," *Huberman Lab* podcast, August 21, 2022, www.hubermanlab.com/episode/what-alcohol-does-to-your-body-brain-health.
5. Tim Jewell, "Taking Melatonin: Can You Mix Melatonin and Alcohol?," Healthline, updated April 29, 2023, www.healthline.com/health/melatonin-and-alcohol#warnings.

DAY EIGHTEEN: BOUNDARIES ARE YOUR BEST FRIEND

1. Nedra Glover Tawwab, *Set Boundaries, Find Peace: A Guide to Reclaiming Yourself* (New York: TarcherPerigee, 2021), 41–42.
2. Annie F. Downs, *Chase the Fun: 100 Days to Discover Fun Right Where You Are* (Grand Rapids, Mich.: Revell, 2022), day 18.

DAY NINETEEN: JOYFUL MOVEMENT

1. *Legally Blonde,* directed by Robert Luketic, featuring Reese Witherspoon, Luke Wilson, Selma Blair, and Matthew Davis (Beverly Hills, Calif.: Metro-Goldwyn-Mayer [MGM], 2001), DVD.
2. Hussain Al-Zubaidi, "Movement Is Medicine," NHS England, November 16, 2022, www.england.nhs.uk/blog/movement-is-medicine.
3. Buddy T, "Chronic Drinking Increases Cortisol Levels," Verywellmind, updated January 22, 2024, www.verywellmind.com/heavy-drinking-increases-stress-hormone-63201.
4. "Exercising to Relax," Harvard Health Publishing, July 7, 2020, www.health.harvard.edu/staying-healthy/exercising-to-relax.

DAY TWENTY: THE POWER OF GRATITUDE

1. Arthur C. Brooks, "How to Be Thankful When You Don't Feel Thankful," *The Atlantic,* November 24, 2021, www.theatlantic.com/family/archive/2021/11/gratitude-thanksgiving/620799.
2. Madhuleena Chowdhury, "The Neuroscience of Gratitude and Effects on the Brain," PositivePsychology.com, April 9, 2019, https://positivepsychology.com/neuroscience-of-gratitude.

DAY TWENTY-ONE: REDEFINING SELF-CARE

1. Amanda E. White, *Not Drinking Tonight: The Workbook; A Clinician's Guide to Helping Clients Examine Their Relationship with Alcohol* (self-pub., CreateSpace, 2016), 91.
2. Genesis 2:2–3.

DAY TWENTY-TWO: NEW WAYS TO COPE

1. Ann Voskamp, *WayMaker: Finding the Way to the Life You've Always Dreamed Of* (Nashville, Tenn.: W Publishing Group, 2022), 197.

DAY TWENTY-FIVE: JESUS AND WINE

1. Scott J. Shifferd, "What Kind of Wine Did Jesus Drink?," The Breath of God, https://godsbreath.net/2011/05/20/did-jesus-drink-wine/comment-page-12.
2. "Units in Calories and Wine," Drinkaware, March 8, 2023, www.drinkaware.co.uk/facts/alcoholic-drinks-and-units/units-and-calories-in-alcoholic-drinks/wine.
3. Ryan Hasty, "Wine in the Bible: Fermented Wine," University Church of Christ, April 14, 2016, www.auchurch.com/resources/articles/2016/04/14/wine-in-the-bible-fermented-wine.
4. Exodus 20:3.

DAY TWENTY-SIX: THE SCIENCE OF JOY

1. Anushree Karkhanis and Ream Al-Hasani, "Dynorphin and Its Role in Alcohol Use Disorder," *Brain Research* 1735 (March 2020): 146742, https://doi.org/10.1016/j.brainres.2020.146742.
2. Marc A. Schuckit, "Alcohol, Anxiety, and Depressive Disorders," *Alcohol Health and Research World* 20, no. 2 (1996): 81–85, www.ncbi.nlm.nih.gov/pmc/articles/PMC6876499.
3. Amy Keller, "Alcohol and Dopamine," DrugRehab.com, updated March 20, 2023, www.drugrehab.com/addiction/alcohol/alcoholism/alcohol-and-dopamine.

DAY TWENTY-SEVEN: ALCOHOL AND ANXIETY

1. Y-L Lu and H. N. Richardson, "Alcohol, Stress Hormones, and the Prefrontal Cortex: A Proposed Pathway to the Dark Side of Addiction," *Neuroscience* 277 (July 2014): 139–51, https://doi.org/10.1016/j.neuroscience.2014.06.053.
2. Buddy T, "Chronic Drinking Increases Cortisol Levels," Verywellmind, updated January 22, 2024, www.verywellmind.com/heavy-drinking-increases-stress-hormone-63201.
3. Kenneth Abernathy, L. Judson Chandler, and John J. Woodward, "Alcohol and the Prefrontal Cortex," *International Review of Neurobiology* 91 (2010): 289–320, https://doi.org/10.1016/S0074-7742(10)91009-X.
4. Jeremiah 29:11.

DAY TWENTY-EIGHT: RENEWING YOUR CONFIDENCE

1. "Train the Brain Effectively Using Visualization," Neuro11, accessed April 8, 2024, https://neuro11.de/principles/train-the-brain-effectively-using-visualization.

DAY TWENTY-NINE: THE HIDDEN DANGERS OF ALCOHOL

1. IARC Working Group on the Evaluation of Carcinogenic Risks to Humans, "Alcohol Drinking," *IARC Monographs on the Evaluation of Carcinogenic Risks to Humans* 44 (1988): 3, www.ncbi.nlm.nih.gov/books/NBK531662.
2. Samir Zakhari, "Overview: How Is Alcohol Metabolized by the Body?," *Alcohol Research and Health* 29, no. 4 (2006): 245–54, www.ncbi.nlm.nih.gov/pmc/articles/PMC6527027.
3. "Known and Probable Human Carcinogens," American Cancer Society, July 8, 2022, www.cancer.org/cancer/risk-prevention/understanding-cancer-risk/known-and-probable-human-carcinogens.html.
4. Sandee LaMotte, "Pandemic Fueled Alcohol Abuse, Especially Among Women, but There Are Treatment Options," *CNN,* December 18, 2022, https://edition.cnn.com/2022/12/18/health/alcohol-treatment-options-lisa-ling-wellness/index.html; quoting from *This Is Life with Lisa Ling,* season 9, episode 5, "We Have a Drinking Problem," produced by Lisa Ling, aired December 18, 2022, on CNN.
5. George Cholankeril et al., "Impact of COVID-19 Pandemic on Liver Transplantation and Alcohol-Associated Liver Disease in the USA," *Hepatology* 74, no. 6 (December 2021): 3316–29, www.ncbi.nlm.nih.gov/pmc/articles/PMC8426752.
6. Jovan Julien, Turgay Ayer, Elliot B. Tapper, Jagpreet Chhatwal, "The Rising Costs of Alcohol-Associated Liver Disease in the United States," abstract, *The American Journal of Gastroenterology* 119, no. 2 (February 2024): 270–77, https://doi.org/10.14309/ajg.0000000000002405.
7. Karla Adkins, "From Happy Hour to ICU: What Happened After Karla Adkins Found Out She Was in Liver Failure at 37?," *"But Jesus Drank Wine" & Other Stories that Kept Us Stuck* podcast, hosted by Christy Osborne and Meade Holland Shirley, episode 27, June 2023, https://open.spotify.com/episode/5HH57G4vAqy1lnnZRkX3jN.
8. Paul G. Thomes et al., "Natural Recovery by the Liver and Other Or-

gans After Chronic Alcohol Use," *Alcohol Research* 41, no. 1 (April 2021), https://doi.org/10.35946/arcr.v41.1.05.

9. American Heart Association News, "Drinking Red Wine for Heart Health? Read This Before You Toast," American Heart Association, May 24, 2019, www.heart.org/en/news/2019/05/24/drinking-red-wine-for-heart-health-read-this-before-you-toast.
10. "The Impact of Alcohol Consumption on Cardiovascular Health," World Heart Federation, January 20, 2022, https://world-heart-federation.org/news/no-amount-of-alcohol-is-good-for-the-heart-says-world-heart-federation.
11. "Impact of Alcohol Consumption."
12. Elizabeth Fernandez, "Alcohol Can Cause Immediate Risk of Atrial Fibrillation," University of California, San Francisco, August 30, 2021, www.ucsf.edu/news/2021/08/421341/alcohol-can-cause-immediate-risk-atrial-fibrillation.
13. "Alcohol and Cancer Risk," National Cancer Institute, updated July 14, 2021, www.cancer.gov/about-cancer/causes-prevention/risk/alcohol/alcohol-fact-sheet.
14. "Drinking Alcohol," Breastcancer.org, October 12, 2023, www.breastcancer.org/risk/risk-factors/drinking-alcohol.
15. "How Does Alcohol Cause Cancer?," Cancer Research UK, September 1, 2023, www.cancerresearchuk.org/about-cancer/causes-of-cancer/alcohol-and-cancer/how-does-alcohol-cause-cancer.
16. Rebecca Strong, "The Alcoholic Drinks Most Likely to Cause Bloating, Gas, and Acid Reflux, and What to Sip Instead," Business Insider, August 26, 2022, www.businessinsider.com/guides/health/diet-nutrition/which-alcohol-is-not-bad-for-stomach.
17. Molly Smith, "Turns Out Your 'Gut Feelings' Are Real. How Gut and Mental Health are Connected," Loma Linda University Health, July 19, 2023, https://news.llu.edu/health-wellness/turns-out-your-gut-feelings-are-real-how-gut-and-mental-health-are-connected.

DAY THIRTY: WELLNESS IN DISGUISE

1. drinkavaline.com.
2. drinkmomwater.com.
3. "Alcohol and Breast Cancer Risk," Breast Cancer Now, https://breast

cancernow.org/about-breast-cancer/awareness/breast-cancer-causes/alcohol-and-breast-cancer-risk.

4. Holly Honderich, "What's Behind Canada's Drastic New Alcohol Guidance," *BBC News,* January 18, 2023, www.bbc.com/news/world-us-canada-64311705.
5. "What's in the Bottle: Ireland Leads the Way as the First Country in the EU to Introduce Comprehensive Health Labelling of Alcohol Products," World Health Organization, May 26, 2023, www.who.int/europe/news/item/26-05-2023-what-s-in-the-bottle--ireland-leads-the-way-as-the-first-country-in-the-eu-to-introduce-comprehensive-health-labelling-of-alcohol-products.
6. Anna H. Grummon and Marissa G. Hall, "Updated Health Warnings for Alcohol—Informing Consumers and Reducing Harm," *The New England Journal of Medicine* 387, no. 9 (August 27, 2022): 772–74, www.nejm.org/doi/full/10.1056/NEJMp2206494.

DAY THIRTY-ONE: REDEFINING FUN

1. C. S. Lewis, *Reflections on the Psalms* (New York: Harcourt, Brace, 1958), 93–97.

DAY THIRTY-TWO: FILLING THE GAP AND EMBRACING OUR EMOTIONS

1. Jennie Allen, *Get Out of Your Head Study Guide: A Study in Philippians* (Grand Rapids, Mich.: Zondervan, 2020), 88.
2. Bryan E. Robinson, "The 90-Second Rule That Builds Self-Control," Psychology Today, April 26, 2020, www.psychologytoday.com/us/blog/the-right-mindset/202004/the-90-second-rule-builds-self-control.
3. Asmir Gračanin, Lauren M. Bylsma, Ad J. J. M. Vingerhoets, "Is Crying a Self-Soothing Behavior?," *Frontiers in Psychology* 5 (May 2014), https://doi.org/10.3389/fpsyg.2014.00502.

DAY THIRTY-THREE: VALUES REKINDLED

1. Ann Voskamp, *WayMaker: Finding the Way to the Life You've Always Dreamed Of* (Nashville, Tenn.: W Publishing Group, 2022), 17.

DAY THIRTY-FIVE: ALCOHOL AND THE OFFICE

1. *Friends,* season 5, episode 18, "The One Where Rachel Smokes," directed by Todd Holland, written by David Crane, Marta Kauffman, and Michael Curtis, featuring Jennifer Aniston, aired April 8, 1999, on NBC.
2. Ian Parsley et al., "Association Between Workplace Absenteeism and Alcohol Use Disorder from the National Survey on Drug Use and Health, 2015–2019," *JAMA Network Open* 5, no. 3 (March 2022): e222954, https://jamanetwork.com/journals/jamanetworkopen/fullarticle/2790205.
3. Ruth Weissenborn and Theodore Duka, "Acute Alcohol Effects on Cognitive Function in Social Drinkers: Their Relationship to Drinking Habits," *Psychopharmacology* 165 (January 2003): 306–312.
4. Aaron M. White, "What Happened? Alcohol, Memory Blackouts, and the Brain," *Alcohol Research and Health* 27, no. 2 (2003): 186–96, www.ncbi.nlm.nih.gov/pmc/articles/PMC6668891.

DAY THIRTY-SIX: BREAKING THE CHAINS OF SHAME

1. Curt Thompson, *The Soul of Shame: Retelling the Stories We Believe About Ourselves* (Downers Grove, Ill.: InterVarsity Press, 2015), 67.
2. Jess Connolly, *You Are the Girl for the Job: Daring to Believe the God Who Calls You* (Grand Rapids, Mich.: Zondervan, 2019), 119.

DAY THIRTY-SEVEN: SOBERING UP TO MOMMY WINE CULTURE

1. Frances Mulraney, "Tropicana Apologizes for Celebrity Ad Campaign Showing Celebrity Parents Sneaking Mimosas from Secret Refrigerators Because Twitter Decided It Was 'Demeaning to Moms and Fueled Alcoholism,'" DailyMail.com, December 17, 2020, www.dailymail.co.uk/news/article-9063849/Tropicana-apologizes-ad-campaign-suggested-alcohol-answer-stressed-parents.html.
2. Irina Gonzalez, "Here's Exactly What's Wrong with Mommy Wine Culture," *Good Housekeeping,* September 29, 2001, www.goodhousekeeping.com/life/parenting/a34655653/wine-mom-jokes-danger.
3. Lauren Sausser, "More Women Are Drinking Themselves Sick. The Biden Administration Is Concerned," March 21, 2024, *CBS News,* www

.cbsnews.com/news/women-drinking-alcohol-health-problems-biden-administration-response.

4. Gonzalez, "Mommy Wine Culture."
5. Gina Wynn (@whitegrapesandinshape), "Don't act like you've never done it. I mean if I'm gonna stand outside in 30 degree temps . . ." Instagram video, February 3, 2023, www.instagram.com/reel/CoM51f5OMuD/?igsh=MWp3NTg2MnNINmZ3Mg.
6. "Deaths Attributed to Tobacco, Alcohol and Drugs, World, 2019," Our World in Data, https://ourworldindata.org/grapher/substances-risk-factor-vs-direct-deaths.

DAY THIRTY-EIGHT: TRAVEL AND VACATIONS WITHOUT ALCOHOL

1. "How Airplane Travel Affects Your Body," Cleveland Clinic, October 19, 2023, https://health.clevelandclinic.org/dehydration-exhaustion-and-gas-what-flying-on-an-airplane-does-to-your-body.

DAY FORTY: REFLECTIONS ON THE JOURNEY

1. John J. Skowronski, W. Richard Walker, Dawn X. Henderson, and Gary D. Bond, "Chapter Three—The Fading Affect Bias: Its History, Its Implications, and Its Future," abstract, *Advances in Experimental Social Psychology* 49, (2014): 163–218, https://doi.org/10.1016/B978-0-12-800052-6.00003-2.

About the Author

Christy Osborne, raised in Los Angeles, graduated from the University of Southern California and Pepperdine University School of Law. After passing the California bar exam, she relocated to London and assumed roles in law, public relations, and business development. She worked for the UK Parliament and founded a popular website for American expat women. Christy found her true calling when she chose sobriety and discovered a passion for helping women with their own journeys. A highly trained senior sobriety coach, she empowers women in the United States and United Kingdom to redefine their relationships with alcohol. She lives with her husband and two children, Ella and Carter, and their cavapoo, Copper, in London.

About the Type

This book was set in Bembo, a typeface based on an old-style Roman face that was used for Cardinal Pietro Bembo's tract *De Aetna* in 1495. Bembo was cut by Francesco Griffo (1450–1518) in the early sixteenth century for Italian Renaissance printer and publisher Aldus Manutius (1449–1515). The Lanston Monotype Company of Philadelphia brought the well-proportioned letterforms of Bembo to the United States in the 1930s.